Praise fo

MW00696315

"*Kiss and Tell* does what no other book on the subject of sex has done—it sits you down at the kitchen table with real women of all ages as they tell you their stories—of their first times, their secret desires, what they wish their partners would do, or not do, or do again. The women of *Kiss and Tell* are alternately poignant, frank, lusty and funny—and they are, to a woman, breathtakingly honest. As you read about their sexual desires, you are bound to find out more about your own."

—SARAH BIRD, AUTHOR OF *THE GAP YEAR*
AND *THE FLAMENCO ACADEMY*

"*As a journalist and writer obsessed by everyday American lifestyles, I've always wanted to know more about the two biggies you're never supposed to ask about: money and sex. By combining the powers of thoughtful, open-minded journalism and empathetic medical expertise, Anne Rodgers and Dr. Maureen Whelihan have accomplished what other clinicians and sex studies couldn't do. They have uncorked fascinating anecdotes from the epic, lifelong story of female sexual experiences. Kiss and Tell is a surprising, heartfelt and valuable book.*"

—HANK STUEVER, AUTHOR OF *TINSEL: A SEARCH
FOR AMERICA'S CHRISTMAS PRESENT*

"*It's hard to overestimate the importance of dialogue when it comes to the subject of passion and desire. Men need and want this information, which Kiss and Tell cheerfully provides through its sensual, eye opening stories.*"

—CHRISTOPHER KENNEDY LAWFORD, AUTHOR OF
RECOVER TO LIVE AND *MOMENTS OF CLARITY*

"Not only will this book answer many questions, but it will also empower more women (and men) to ask the appropriate questions of their healthcare providers and get the dialogue going to help us all enjoy the sex we want. More importantly, it will help reassure lay people that 'normal' can mean many different things to many different people. The open-ended responses to this survey are the best sex education available today."

—ALAN M. ALTMAN MD, PAST PRESIDENT, INTERNATIONAL SOCIETY FOR THE STUDY OF WOMEN'S SEXUAL HEALTH AND AUTHOR OF *MAKING LOVE THE WAY WE USED TO . . . OR BETTER: THE SECRETS TO SATISFYING MIDLIFE SEXUALITY*

"Sigmund Freud famously asked the question, 'What do women want?' Now Anne Rodgers and Dr. Maureen Whelihan have given us a definitive series of answers from women in all stages of life that are sometimes startling and often surprising. Not only do we learn what women want, we find out what they actually do . . . and don't do. And why or why not. If Freud had had this book, he wouldn't have been so confused!"

—SCOTT EYMAN, BIOGRAPHER OF *LION OF HOLLYWOOD* AND *EMPIRE OF DREAMS*

Kiss and Tell

Secrets of Sexual Desire
from Women 15 to 97

Anne Rodgers with
Maureen Whelihan MD

Published by Soft Spot Press

ISBN: 978-0-9885331-0-3

Printed in the United States of America

10 9 8 7 6 5 4 3 2 1

CONTENTS

Kiss and Tell is based on a survey of 1,300 women (and follow-up interviews with almost 100 of them) who were bold enough to tell the truth about the elusive nature of their sexual desire: what inspires it, what diminishes it and what keeps it alive decade after decade.

INTRODUCTION

KISS AND TELL IMPARTS A REASSURING TRUTH ABOUT SEX FOR all women to take away: *You are normal.*

Sadly, this is an affirmation many women have trouble internalizing, perhaps because we're all just a little bit worried that *our* insecurities and *our* preferences are just a little bit, well, odd.

The veil of secrecy that still exists when it comes to talking about sex doesn't help. Even close girlfriends tend to keep bedroom matters private. They'll crack a joke, sure, or tell an occasional story, but genuine sharing about what goes on sexually with their partners isn't an integral part of most female friendships, despite what *Sex and the City* would have us believe.

So it's a bit revolutionary to push past the focus on bedroom techniques, positions and partners—and delve deeper to the core issue of desire.

After years of medical study, client confidentialities and observation of patients, gynecologist and sex educator Dr.

Maureen Whelihan is confident when she pronounces, "Women don't have low desire for sex; they have low desire for the sex they're having."

And that's a shame. Because sex matters.

It matters when you're having good sex and it matters when you're having bad sex. And don't kid yourself: Which one you're having has a huge impact on your quality of life.

Desire is critical for good sex, and for women, that factor is elusive. Desire seems to come and go of its own accord; it can feel ephemeral to a woman, often difficult to conjure at the moment it's needed—and sometimes altogether invisible.

Men rarely suffer this fate: They have the advantage of higher levels of testosterone, which keeps their desire on a more even keel, and much closer to the surface than it is for women, equipped as we are with the more docile hormone estrogen.

Without a raging hormone, a woman's sexual desire is subject to a host of influences, including but hardly limited to the cleanliness of her house, the proximity of her children, the smell of her partner, the length of her to-do list, her worry of pregnancy, her fatigue, the mood of her boss that day at work, resentments toward her partner, her perception of her body, her feelings of being loved, the time of the month, psychological issues from her previous sexual partner and literally hundreds of other concerns. For the vast majority of women, such issues are perfectly capable of crowding out our biological desire for sex.

If there's one thing our survey proves, it's that a woman's desire for sex is a multifaceted and fragile thing, which is why the subject should be front and center in any conversation about a satisfying sex life.

AN UNLIKELY BEGINNING

It all started with a toothbrush.

A FAITHFUL READER CALLED ONE DAY TO ENCOURAGE ME TO write a newspaper story about her gynecologist's practice of recommending a low-cost, battery-powered toothbrush to her older patients as a vibrator substitute.

At the time, my designated beat was women over 45, so naturally I was shocked and delighted at such a titillating story. I looked up the unconventional Dr. Whelihan to ask whether she was indeed recommending toothbrushes in this way.

"Why not?" she asked me, with nary a hint of self-consciousness. "As women age, they often need more direct clitoral stimulation to achieve orgasm. The frequency is similar to that of a vibrator, and it's discreet and quiet. Just don't use the brush side!"

The good doctor happened to stumble on this innovative idea through her visionary husband, who one day was using a battery powered toothbrush for its intended purpose. The thought occurred to him that the vibration he was feeling in his hand might be better enjoyed at a different location.

He excitedly informed Maureen of his discovery that night, and the doc—always intrigued by . . . ahem . . . research of this nature—was more than willing to see what the buzz was all about.

Her verdict? "Holy smokes! Talk about a quickie!"

Professionally, she immediately saw the battery powered toothbrushes wider potential.

"How can you beat this new sex toy that is effective, inexpensive and discreet?" she says.

Soon Dr. Whelihan was recommending it at the office to older patients who seemed likely candidates, such as women complaining of difficulty reaching orgasm or simply those wanting an inexpensive way to try a vibrator. A toothbrush is discreet as well, and her clients who traveled frequently told Dr. Whelihan they were relieved that a large and potentially embarrassing vibrator wasn't going to be scanned during a luggage check. Teenagers living at home liked the tool's innocent exterior as well.

That story led to another, as Dr. Whelihan and I realized we were both intrigued by the ups and downs of midlife women's sex drives, as well as the intensely unique nature of each woman's desire. We began talking about how age and experience affect a woman's drive and libido.

From her practice, Dr. Whelihan knows that even when women are not getting the sex they want or need, many still have an immense desire for great sex. We began to wonder what role desire plays in a couple's lives, and what factors most affect a woman's libido throughout her lifetime.

So we created an informal survey to gather data directly from women—specifically the South Florida suburbia patients in Dr. Whelihan's gynecological practice.

We asked six questions:

1. What stimulates your desire?
2. What's in your brain during sex? (What are you thinking about?)

3. What is your quickest route to orgasm?
4. Describe the best sex of your life. How old [were you] and why?
5. What is the one thing you wish your partner would *not* do in regard to sex?
6. What is the biggest lie you were told about sex?

The questions were worded specifically to elicit information about desire, arousal and preferences. Our open-ended queries meant no two women's responses were identical, which was both exhilarating and a statistical nightmare. (In such a format, no one response garners an overwhelming percentage of the total.)

Our survey differs from those that have gone before by zeroing in on women's desire. That's because all the how-to books in the world don't do much good if a woman isn't in the mood to experiment, relax, slow down and focus on her pleasure—all of which she's unlikely to do without desire.

Patients were offered our survey in the privacy of their exam room at Dr. Whelihan's office. Many were not just interested, but flattered to be asked for input. Frequently, the survey takers initiated a broader discussion about sex once the doctor arrived.

"My patients wanted to provide their feedback for other women to compare themselves to or relate to," says Dr. Whelihan. "They felt they had great ideas to offer, and they trusted us that this was a confidential endeavor."

Eventually, 1,300 women—ages 15 to 97—completed the survey. Each one signed a waiver; we granted them anonymity in exchange for complete honesty, and their authentic answers are our reward. Freed of consequences, our survey participants responded with gratifying candor. *Kiss and Tell's* survey tapped women's willingness to open up about all manner of bedroom issues—and readers will be heartened to see how quickly they begin to feel normal as the vast array of other women's experiences unfold.

Once the survey results were tallied, I conducted in-depth, face-to-face interviews with a diverse sampling of women—straight, lesbian, married, bisexual, widowed, single and divorced.

Our respondents were eager to share information that might educate others or shed light on the mysterious subject of sexual desire and how it waxes and wanes throughout a woman's life.

Women don't routinely have such intimate conversations—even with a lifelong friend—for a variety of reasons. Pouring out one's bedroom secrets carries the risk of feeling like a betrayal of the private bond a woman shares with her partner or husband, not to mention the possibility of experiencing disapproval or judgment from the friend.

Though younger women are a bit more open to discussing sex with their friends, we found women over 40 rarely express their fears, desires and insecurities in this intensely personal realm. When such confidences might expose an inadequacy or a problem a woman is experiencing with her lover, the chances of sharing drop even further.

Our goal with *Kiss and Tell* is to allay that sense of isolation through our wide and colorful group of outspoken subjects. Within these real-life stories, every woman is sure to find a reflection of herself—and reassurance of her own normalcy.

As the in-depth interviews unfolded, I became absorbed by the rich detail we were collecting, while Dr. Whelihan was intent on discovering answers that could lead to the betterment of all sexual relationships. Getting at the truth behind women's elusive desire for sex became our obsession.

So we set out to examine the unpredictable nature of

women's sexual desire, to find the trends within each decade of a woman's life and get an honest look at the true nature of female desire. We're glad you're along for the ride.

MEET THE DOCTOR

THE OFFICE OF DR. MAUREEN WHELIHAN—A.K.A. DR. MO—
isn't fancy. It's not part of a large medical complex or even a
medium-size office building. It's a small, one-story structure
on a fairly busy corner in the South Florida community of Wel-
lington.

Parking can be tricky some days, because two other doctors
share the space, but if you're lucky, you'll score a shady spot.
Inside, the space is spotless and modest. The vibe is friendly,
caring and professional. Dr. Mo sports stylish heels, but never a
white coat. Staff members refer to everyone as "sugar," "sweetie"
or "mama." When I drop by for quick fact checks, I leave feeling
cocooned and cared for—and I'm not even a patient.

From this setting come the first stories Dr. Mo tells me
about her practice. They are detail-rich, sometimes shocking
and always fascinating, allowing me an intriguing glimpse into
the private world of female sexuality (with no breach of patient
confidentiality). The stories illuminate the things women are
willing to share with their physician—*if* that doctor is comfortable enough to query the patient about her sex life. By opening
wide the door for communication in this still-sensitive area, Dr.
Mo knows she has found her true calling.

How do such intimate, closed-door conversations begin?

For starters, each new patient fills out a questionnaire, which includes a query about sexual activity. Then Dr. Whelihan follows up in person, with her long-standing routine of asking each woman face-to-face about the quality of her sex life. Since national studies show that a third of younger women and half of older women say they have problems with sex (such as lack of desire, pain during intercourse or inability to achieve orgasm), this would seem to be a natural topic of conversation between doctor and patient.

Sadly, it is not.

A recent survey of 1,154 gynecologists published in the *Journal of Sexual Medicine*[1] shows less than 14 percent ask their patients about pleasure with sexual activity.

At Dr. Whelihan's office, patients usually are glad for the opportunity to have a straightforward conversation about sex with a nonjudgmental listener. Most jump right in.

If a patient answers no, she's not having sex, the doc's next question is, "Lack of interest or lack of a partner?" If it's lack of a partner, the doctor admits she can't summon good lovers out of thin air, but she often reminds patients that do-it-yourself sex is always fun too. If the response is lack of interest or a non-functioning partner, Dr. Whelihan stands ready with a handy list of helpful suggestions and treatments for low desire.

With patients who say yes, they're having sex, Dr. Whelihan asks whether they're having orgasms. Answer yes to this one and the doc is content. But a negative response to this personal question elicits a discussion about what might be preventing the patient from achieving the pleasure she deserves. And thus the

---

1   "What We Don't Talk About When We Don't Talk About Sex: Results of a National Survey of U.S. Obstetritian/Gynecologists," from *The Journal of Sexual Medicine* (May 2012, Vol. 5, Issue 5),

conversation continues.

With her frank and engaging manner, Dr. Whelihan elicits copious amounts of information during such exchanges. Most patients are relieved to finally have a healthy talk about something that matters very deeply to them, but is so often off-limits.

Dr. Mo believes that enhancing her patients' sex lives is a critical part of her job, but many gynecologists are reluctant to interrogate their patients about something so intimate. Male doctors especially may have trouble negotiating the line between concerned professional and sounding like a closet pervert when they bring up the subject of orgasms with female patients.

WHY DON'T MORE GYNs TALK TO US ABOUT SEX?

One solution that would address doctors' reticence to open conversations about sex is to offer professionals additional education. Medical school training is shamefully inadequate at preparing gynecologists—of either gender—to navigate this sensitive territory. A study of medical school curricula in North America as detailed in the *International Journal of Impotence Research*[2] reports that 61 percent of schools offer less than ten hours (total) of study in sexual health. This barely covers the anatomy, much less the psychological aspects of approaching patients about sexuality. No wonder so many doctors are tongue-tied!

The study also showed that only 15 percent of *all* medical schools offer greater than 20 hours of sex education during a four-year program.

---

2   "The Human Sexuality Education of Physicians in North American Medical Schools," from *International Journal of Impotence Research* (2003) 15, Suppl 5, S41–S45. doi:10.1038/sj.ijir.3901071

The result is a gynecological community permeated with individuals who bring their own particular inhibitions to their practices, and who too often lack the training that would allow them to speak casually, confidently and without judgment to their clients about sex.

In fact, throughout history, there has been no encouragement from the medical profession for women to embrace the sexual nature of their vaginas. In earlier times, when doctors were exclusively male, there was for all intents and purposes a ban against even acknowledging the vagina as a sex organ.

Today's attitudes have evolved much less than one would expect. From a girl's first visit, she learns that gynecologists invariably focus on the reproductive aspects of her genitalia. The folks in the white coats are comfortable talking about the cervix, but not the clitoris; happy to discuss yeast infections but loath to mention orgasms. Too often they are quick to order tests but slow to open a conversation about the raging hormones of a teenager. As a result, females of all ages receive minimal input from an educated professional as to the pleasure that might proceed from understanding how their bodies respond to various stimuli.

So women get the message loud and clear: A vagina is a place to have a baby or an infection, not an orgasm.

Fortunately, through events that occurred early in her career, Dr. Mo was able to overcome institutional barriers and gain a wider knowledge of sexual health. Credit her curiosity, a bit of trial-and-error and a 32-year-old man who knew he was really a woman.

Around 1994, as a second-year resident at the University of Florida, Shands Jacksonville, Dr. Whelihan's natural inquisitiveness led to her first attempt at asking a patient about sex. Her initial effort fell flat.

"Unfortunately it was a 'closed' question," she admits. "I said to a 54-year-old patient—I was 20 years her junior—'So, you're not having sex, right?' And her response was, 'Of course I am, dear!' Note to self—*wrong* approach."

So she learned. She quit making assumptions and began listening with an open attitude. And when the opportunity arose to do pre-op work with the aforementioned transsexual, who was reassigning from male to female, Dr. Mo was the only resident in the department willing to step up. So in 1996, she became the primary surgeon (working under a mentor) for the patient's orchiectomy (removal of the testes), which is part one of gender reassignment surgery. And from that time on, she found human sexuality fascinating.

So much so that in 2002 she opted out of the baby-delivery business.

"If you're not doing obstetrics, it's much easier to explore the sexuality of patients," says Dr. Mo. "There's more time, the patients are older and are generally more willing to engage."

It was when she began focusing exclusively on gynecology that Dr. Whelihan added the question, "Are you sexually active?" to her office intake form. And in 2004, she began consciously following up in person with specific queries.

For all the information and health advice she's given out over the years, it's safe to say Dr. Mo has learned even more than her patients. Despite her open mind, they're able to confound her notions and expectations time and again.

There's the widow in her eighties who recently experienced her first orgasm and is now having the best sex of her life. And the sexually active teenager hoping for an elusive orgasm who nervously giggled her way through a short anatomy lesson from the doctor. And the patient in her seventies with the perfectly coiffed white hair that looks like it's done professionally every week—and who is the subject of a story Dr. Whelihan loves to tell.

"If you had to guess, based on her appearance and personality, you'd say she was maybe a retired librarian," says Dr. Mo, who noted during the exam that the patient's vulvar tissue was "healthy, lubricated and very youthful in appearance."

A glance at the woman's medical chart indicated the patient wasn't using any estrogen products.

Like every other med student, Dr. Whelihan had seen the literature indicating that if you can have three orgasms a week, you can maintain a healthy, youthful vagina into late life. The textbooks insist that regular orgasms keep the vagina healthy—which means supple, pink, juicy and vital.

"So in the exam room, I look and see the picture-perfect healthy vagina!" says Dr. Mo. "I had to know if the textbooks were true."

So she asks the patient if she's sexually active. The answer is affirmative, accompanied by a small smile.

"Are you by any chance having sex three times a week?" was Dr. Mo's next query.

"Yes, dear, but you're asking a lot of questions," said the patient.

"One more: Do you have orgasms every time?" asked Dr. Mo, who was closing in on the proof she sought.

"Yes, but why do you care?" said the patient, amused.

Dr. Whelihan explained that she'd read studies maintaining that regular orgasms could assure vaginal health (since they increase blood flow and hormones to the region), but that this was the first time she'd ever been able to put it together.

"The patient's confident nod let me know I wasn't telling her anything she hadn't figured out on her own, but she indicated she couldn't wait to go home and share the info with her hubby."

Being willing to have such conversations brings its own set of surprises. When the survey for this book was under way, Dr. Whelihan would occasionally glance at a patient's answers as they handed the form to her in the exam room. If questions were left blank, and an opportunity arose, she might press for a response to help complete the page.

When she noticed that numerous women said the one thing they wish their partner wouldn't do in bed was talk, she created opportunities during the exam to seek clarification. She learned that while a ration of compliments is rarely frowned upon, many women do *not* welcome constant chatter or a barrage of questions. (Worse yet is a man who's narrating *his* fantasy, ignorant of the fact that his partner may be lost in her own scenario.)

"One 40-something patient who wrote that she just wanted her husband to be quiet during sex told me during her office visit that she finally ended up saying to him: 'Stop talking! I'm trying to have a fantasy and you're *not in it!*'"

While her patients like how easy it is to share their deepest desires and sexual concerns with Dr. Whelihan, more traditional gynecological health concerns naturally constitute a large part of her patient interaction.

On their surveys, some women mention serious health issues that had an impact on their libido. But it's not just disease that shoulders out the desire for sex in women's everyday lives—it's also mundane things, such as being overweight or getting older.

SHE'S NOT HEAVY, SHE'S MY LOVER

"I have many voluptuous patients who are perfectly happy to

get naked with no inhibition," says Dr. Mo, "but others cite weight as a significant barrier to their willingness to be nude in the bedroom.

"It's one of the most common complaints I hear. Women say they don't want to undress because they are too fat, too gross, too self-conscious, too whatever. This libido issue is *totally* up to us to change—and *can* be corrected," says the doctor, who took her own advice last year and reached her goal of losing 30 pounds. "What we put in our mouths is absolutely up to us . . . no excuses."

"That said, I often tell my patients that men are shallow creatures; when it comes to sex, they just want to see you naked, all of you, because men are greatly aroused with visual stimuli. In an amorous frame of mind, they are not seeing the pockets of cellulite you're obsessing over, or the twenty pounds you've put on since the wedding. They see *sex*! So if a patient isn't willing to diet and change the situation, then I tell them to stop using the 'I'm too heavy' excuse as a dodge, and remember that your lover is usually much less judgmental than you!"

CARBS CAN CROWD OUT SEX

Dr. Whelihan mentions another tie-in between sex and excessive consumption—especially of sugar.

"Sugars—carbohydrates—stimulate the serotonin in the brain and satisfy the pleasure center," she says. "But sex also satisfies the pleasure center, so if you keep hitting it with sugar instead, you can decrease the desire for sex.

"While women think that in their early weight-loss phases it's 'feeling skinny' that makes them want more sex, I would argue that it is the restriction of carbohydrates and sugars that is really what is making your brain crave sex."

Keep in mind, she adds, a too-full belly causes most people's libido to drop. If serotonin is elevated through food, it sends an inhibitory message to the pleasure center. In addition, your blood flow is now concentrated in your stomach, trying to digest food. Consequently, it's being diverted from the genitalia, making arousal difficult in both men and women. Simple changes—such as eating less—can cause an increase in sexual interest within days.

"And weight loss will be close behind in weeks or months," she assures her patients.

DECLINING ESTROGEN

Another common complaint heard in Dr. Whelihan's office relating to desire is that a hysterectomy has caused a severe drop in a patient's passion.

While a woman may blame the hysterectomy, it's the removal of the ovaries that is the culprit, says the doctor, since ovaries are responsible for all of our estrogen and half our testosterone. If they're removed—especially prematurely—sex drive can definitely be affected.

"These are the sex hormones which provide an excitatory stimulus to the pleasure center, so naturally, without them, desire can diminish," says Dr. Mo.

With appropriate hormone therapy, libido in women without ovaries can be enhanced, she says, but it often requires much trial and error to achieve the correct combination and dosage.

Dr. Whelihan favors transdermal estradiol—literally "through the skin" methods such as patches, rings, gels or lotions—over oral estrogens, because oral estrogens may block the activity of what little testosterone is still being produced naturally.

If a hysterectomy is performed but the ovaries are left in place and the patient *still* complains of low libido, Dr. Mo asks whether pain is occurring during deep penetration. If so, this can be caused by either a fallopian tube or the ovaries becoming stuck to the vaginal cuff as scar tissue forms during the healing process.

"But sometimes the loss of the uterus is not the real culprit," notes Dr. Whelihan. "The culprit is the underlying issue of loss of fertility, the ability to bear children. Some patients feel like less of a woman when this occurs, and psychological complications from these feelings may lead them to shun sex."

SEX LIVES AFTER 60 . . . AND 70

Since overall the health and sexuality of the aging boomer population is being extended, doctors are dealing with a corresponding increase nationwide—reported by the Centers for Disease Control—of sexually transmitted infections in people over 60.

As an example, Dr. Whelihan recalls an attractive 76-year-old patient who came in for a routine annual exam with no complaints. But a green, frothy discharge was observed, and a vaginal smear revealed trichomoniasis, an STD.

Dr. Mo told the patient both she and her partner needed treatment, but the woman wouldn't accept medication for her partner because she refused to believe he had an infection.

The next day, the woman's granddaughter—who happened to be a nurse—called to ask if Dr. Mo had indeed told her grandmother she had an STD.

Mindful of HIPAA (The Health Insurance Portability and Accountability Act), the doctor asked what the granddaughter had been told. The grandmother had indeed spilled the truth, so Dr. Whelihan confirmed the diagnosis to the nurse.

"I *told* her she needs to be using condoms!" said the granddaughter, laughing in exasperation. "She's got three men she's sleeping with, and she's not sharing that information with any of them!"

"I was thinking the granddaughter would say, 'What kind of quack doctor are you, telling my grandmother she has an STD?' and instead she was scolding her grandmother!"

The take-away here for doctors is to not overlook the possibility of sexually transmitted diseases in the aging patient; for patients, the lesson is to face the risks of unprotected sex, which aren't limited to unwanted pregnancy.

The granddaughter was right to encourage her relative to use condoms. The rising number of STDs in the elderly is attributable to the fact that many men in this age group never wore condoms and don't care to start; and women of this age believe that since they can't get pregnant, condoms aren't necessary.

In fact, the National Institute on Aging reports that people age 50 and older represent almost one-fourth of all people with HIV/AIDS in the United States.[3] Medicare has taken note of this shift and made a step forward in sexual health care by approving payment for STD screenings.

Since seniors aren't chatty in general on the subject of sex, they don't readily talk to their doctors about such issues, and thereby miss the chance to be educated on the importance of protection.

Even couples who agree condoms are a good idea may hesitate to use them for another reason: They can interfere with the man's sexual performance.

"Although an elderly man may have a great erection, he's liable to lose that good boner with the application of a condom," says Dr. Mo. "It presents a dilemma: Good recommendations

---

3   National Institute on Aging. HIV, AIDS, and Older People. Bethesda, MD: U.S. Department of Health and Human Services; 2009.

go against good function at this age."

Her solution is to give prudent advice to the patient, which involves the recommendation for condoms, but to realize the challenges associated with that suggestion.

"I tell them to have a backup plan, which is yearly STD screenings—obviously a distant second," she says.

WHEN IT'S HARD TO GET HARD

No discussion of how medical problems impact women's sexuality is complete without a closer look at how the aging process affects male performance. Men don't have to be seriously ill to experience erectile dysfunction. However, irreversible issues are rare; most ED is preventable and very treatable.

Dr. Whelihan recognizes that some couples are distressed when Viagra, Levitra or Cialis are required for a successful sexual encounter, but she points out that erectile problems due to cardiovascular disease are seen in men in their forties before blood pressure or cholesterol issues even surface.

"As conditions worsen, assistance from the drugs is necessary to get enough blood flow in the penis to allow successful penetration," she says. "This may take a little away from spontaneity, but as we age, this is just one of the things we have to learn to modify."

Dr. Mo emphasizes *prevention* as the main weapon to treat ED, noting that only 15 percent of cases are psychological. The remaining 85 percent are due to physiological (or organic) causes, especially smoking, diabetes and cardiovascular disease.

"The most destructive but preventable disease for erection dysfunction is diabetes," she continues. "Adult-onset diabetes is due to an overconsumption of carbohydrates, so address it now. Patients who tell me that adult-onset diabetes 'runs in the family' are simply telling me that everyone has bad eating habits and does not exercise regularly. Most of the medications folks use are to treat problems they can either prevent or correct with diet and exercise. Stop making excuses!"

If ED is a problem, the doctor recommends a man stop smoking, control his cholesterol via a low-fat diet and get some exercise.

"Keep your sugars down with a low-carbohydrate diet, and exercise. Keep your stress levels under control via exercise or meditation, and manage any high blood pressure early. Notice how many times I said 'diet and exercise'? Don't wait for the condition to occur to make the change, as it may be too late.

"If your doctor—whether urologist, cardiologist or GP—is *not* addressing your sexual concerns, please be the first to raise the question," she urges.

"Nothing is more rewarding than finding a solution for the most private fears a patient has," says Dr. Whelihan. "Discussing sexual concerns can be awkward for some ladies, so much so that they often go years without answers. So how wonderful it is to gain their trust and confidence. I love nothing more than seeing a little kick in a patient's step as we both giggle at the conclusion of the discussion. I have a great job!"

AND THE SURVEY SAYS …

ONE WOMAN WROTE "DON'T TALK DURING SEX" AND ANOTHER wrote "dirty talk makes me hot;" one says "don't rush me" and another says "you're taking too long." Clearly, distilling information about sexual desire from 1,300 women is a study in contrasts.

Dr. Whelihan and I realized early on that since our survey used only open-ended questions (we gave no ready-made responses, no simple boxes to check), we would collect a broad array of answers.

So what did we learn?

First and foremost, kissing is the number one answer for women of all ages when you ask, "What stimulates your desire?" Overall, it's the gold standard for arousing a woman and making her feel receptive. Though teenagers also express a longing for manly lovers, and midlife women very often mention that a glass of wine will put them in the mood, women of all ages cite good kissing most often. (Accordingly, we've devoted a later chapter entirely to this subject.)

As far as alcohol goes, it is women in their forties and fifties who most cite it as a stimulator of desire; the number drops sharply for those in their sixties. While teens may say, "I was really drunk," when describing a sexual encounter, they don't call alcohol a stimulant. However, during in-depth interviews, they often remark that it lowers their inhibitions.

Midlife women gravitate to a cocktail or glass of wine for good reason: They are overwhelmed. They are likely to have teenage children at home; aging parents who might need attention or care; a job with more responsibility than that of a younger woman; and a 20-year marriage to a man they've slept with thousands of times. No wonder these women think to include wine or a cocktail as one of the tools that can banish the day's stresses and lead to a sexual encounter.

As the Decades of Desire chapters unfold, I'll sketch the cultural influences that had an impact on the women of each era, and you'll see how each decade differs from the one before and after. Sometimes, we charted the development *within* a decade as well.

For instance, it is easy to identify that a woman's twenties are a time of transformation. Women I interviewed confirmed significant sexual experimentation during their early twenties, but then expressed consistent satisfaction in their committed relationships by the end of that decade, even admitting relief that the sexual experimentation period was behind them.

Though I intended to interview the women from youngest to oldest, the teenagers proved hard to corral, so while I waited for those meetings to materialize, I began contacting women in the oldest decade. From then on, my process involved seesawing from an older decade to a younger, finally meeting in the middle, to finish off with the fifties.

Unintentionally, this method enabled me to immediately "bookend" the decades, and early on I had a picture of how the youngest respondents stacked up against the oldest.

With an age span of 15 to 97, the great divide is apparent. Women who've been alive almost a century are light-years removed from the straight-talking, sexually experienced—and often empowered—women who represented the teen decade.

One compelling observation resulting from the in-depth interviews succinctly encapsulates the revolution in sexual practices that occurred in the twentieth century: The oldest women, those in their eighties and nineties, told me they lost their virginity anywhere from the age of 23 to 25, while some of our survey's more precocious teens began sexual activity at 14 and 15.

This means an entire decade of life as a virgin (how else to put it?) has been subtracted from today's young women compared with 100 years ago. The early induction to sex for today's girls means what once was a back-burner issue for late teens and 20-somethings is front and center for today's youth.

LESS TALKING, PLEASE

Certain findings from our survey are expected; others are a surprise. A majority of all women said clitoral stimulation is their surest route to orgasm, and since this is hardly a shock to women, we're continually amazed when men find it novel. But Dr. Mo and I were initially puzzled when we read, over and over again, that the one thing women wish their partner would *not* do in regards to sex is talk.

Talk? Really?

Our follow-up interviews made everything clear: Women rate occasional endearments as fine; it's the battery of questions about what feels good, whether his performance is satisfactory or what her requests are that women can do without. Too often it seems this chatter interferes with a woman's ability to concentrate—on either her fantasy or her reality—and thus derails her effort to achieve orgasm.

So, while they hesitate to tell lovers, partners and husbands that mum's the word, given the chance to name their heart's desire, many women said they just wish guys would shut up.

Fantasies, we discovered, are an integral part of a sexual relationship, especially in long-term unions where bedroom doldrums tend to sneak in.

"Fantasies can incorporate thoughts or ideas that are unlikely to occur, but which can stimulate arousal without the risk," says Dr. Whelihan. "They provide a playground for the imagination, where no scenario is off-limits."

And because our brains tend to believe what we tell them, sexy imaginings are an effective tool for turning our thoughts away from household chores and down more erotic pathways.

Some ladies may enjoy narrating their fantasies for a partner; others find such frank communication difficult.

In fact, a good number of surveys indicated that during sex women are thinking about how to wordlessly get their partner to do the right thing. They obviously have misgivings about offering specific direction, perhaps having encountered a partner who resented such tactics, or perhaps just being reticent to voice their desires.

But it would behoove women to speak up in bed, since faking it doesn't assist men in the long run. Dr. Whelihan notes that a good faker just leads a man to believe he's doing it right.

"Men need to understand the difference between groaning—which indicates pleasure—and orgasm, which is rhythmic contractions of the vaginal walls for at least a few seconds," she says.

A CLEAN HOUSE = WILLING PARTNER!

But the issue of satisfaction is entwined with the anatomical differences between men and women, and the reality that orgasms are not a given for women like they are for most men.

Again and again, survey comments show how much effort women are expending in order to achieve orgasm. Answers to the "what's in your brain during sex" question prove that many women feel out of control of their orgasms. They're thinking, "Let it be good this time," or, "Faster ... slower ... up ... down," or, "I want to have an orgasm." It's clear they do not assume success—just as it's clear that men, as they enter into any love-making experience, are definitely assuming success.

Barbara, 33 and married five years, expresses the views of women in this camp.

"They [men] always, always, always, always, always, always have an orgasm." She laughs. "He can be dead asleep and he'll wake up and want to do it when I finish my shower. He'll drive down to Miami in the traffic, get home late and he'll want to do it! It doesn't matter to them!"

She tries to explain why that's so difficult for her.

"When I come into the house and there's crap everywhere and he didn't try to clean up the mess and then at bedtime he wants to get it on, I'm not in the mood. If the house is all tidy, I feel like I can relax. I can't sit and relax in mess and clutter. It's hard enough to relax in bed, and it's harder if I'm thinking about folding the clothes there on the chair. How am I supposed to feel sexual and have that desire when I have tasks and chores smacking me in the face?

"Guys don't think [those things] are even related," Barbara continues. "I hate to make generalizations, but I believe we're more emotional. Two minutes after a fight, he can turn it off. My husband's a wonderful provider and a good man, but it takes me a while to resolve issues after a disagreement. And he'll want to go to bed and have sex. I have to feel at peace to have sex—especially if I'm going to have an orgasm. He says I don't give it up, but in my mind, it's already over with. I'm just saying yes because I don't want to hear him complain that we don't have sex enough. I'm totally not into it. Obviously I don't have an orgasm at those times."

Which leads to another interesting tangent: We found that when women ask, "Where's the Viagra for *me*?" they are actually asking for a pill that enhances their desire.

When men have issues surrounding sex, it almost always involves function. In other words, they have desire, but no ability. Viagra is obviously a pill for function; there's little demand for a supplement to increase male desire for sex (except in cases of depression). Women, who have few issues with function, need a dose of desire—and that's a tougher challenge. The only well-known booster of desire is testosterone, and no FDA-approved version for women is yet available.

One other significant trend we found was that women of all ages say they dislike anal sex. In fact, 12 percent mentioned it as the one thing in regard to sex that they wish their partner would not do. Twelve percent may seem unimpressive, but not for an open-answer survey such as this. Since the format allows for an infinite variety of responses (*everything* is a write-in), it's noteworthy when any answer garners even 10 to 15 percent of the total.

Based on its unpopularity among our respondents, we did in-depth interviews on anal sex, and discovered that the majority of our subjects are rejecting the practice untried; they haven't experimented with anal sex and have decided they don't care to try it. Their reasoning and opinions are explored in detail in a later chapter, along with stories from women who say they find this variation on lovemaking very satisfying.

But first, since 21 percent of our survey participants (almost 300 women) cited kissing as a key element in arousing their passion, let's find out more about this phenomenon.

Why is good kissing a make-or-break deal for so many women?

KISS ME, YOU FOOL

Ask Cathy what constitutes a good kiss and you get quite an education.

"Hmm, well, I think first of all you need to be in the mood," says the 50-year-old mother of two. "There are times when you give the pecks on lips, cheeks, forehead. But that kiss that leads to getting naked . . . it's *so* much more. Firm, not too wet . . . he's kissing my soul. His tongue is moving in and out of my mouth, softly, making me want to open my mouth wider and welcome him in. He alternates between kissing my lips and slipping his tongue in my mouth, taking my breath away. It just totally makes me melt in his arms."

That's the kind of kissing that can change a woman's mind about having sex.

"Kissing is really, really important," states Mia, a 53-year-old divorcée who's been on her own for four years. "If a man isn't a good kisser, I make an automatic assumption that he's not good at everything else. If there's no touch, heat, warmth in the kiss, there's not going to be any anywhere else. So for me [kissing is] a precursor to good sex."

She's not alone. Psychologists at the State University of New York at Albany recently reported that 66 percent of women (and 59 percent of men) had terminated a budding relationship because of a bad kiss.

That's because everyone craves the intimacy that good kissing facilitates.

"The best kiss to make my clothes fall off needs to be confident yet tender and teasing," says Dee, a married, 46-year-old travel consultant. "Mouths barely open, lips and tongue barely touching . . . retreating and then leaning in for more. An occasional nibble on the lips makes me yearn for more. He knows where it's going but doesn't need to say a word."

In *Cherry*, her frank coming-of-age memoir, author Mary Karr lushly describes teenage kissing: "Time will never again stretch to the silky lengths it reaches that spring when you and Phil first sit entangled in his car, the odor of narcissus and jasmine and crab-apple blossoms blowing through the open windows on black wind. Nor will kisses ever again evolve into such baroque forms, delicate as origami in their folds and bendings. . . . He runs his tongue along your lower lip like a question, and you return the inquiry. Then in unison your tongues meet all soft on that same territory and glide together the small distance. Touch and withdraw, taste and test. All the light of your being seems to pour into him at such moments, and his into you."

As Karr writes: "Because the nights don't have sex as an end . . . the kisses are themselves an end."

No less an icon than Albert Einstein has weighed in on the importance of kissing: "Any man who can drive safely while kissing a pretty girl is simply not giving the kiss the attention it deserves," he observed.

Kissing for the sake of kissing is something women of all ages understand, but the sad reality is that—once married—too many men lose touch with the fine art of making out. Their focus narrows down to the goal of intercourse, and kissing is too often treated as a perfunctory prelude.

"I tell guys in my sex lectures to remember back to when they were trying to convince their future wives to have sex with them that very first time," says Dr. Whelihan. "You were trying to convey all your passion and intensity through your kiss, and somehow you communicated your desire, and she responded.

"How many times have you heard a woman say she wasn't planning to go all the way, but the guy was *such* a good kisser?

A CASE IN POINT

Diane met Stu through a mutual friend at dinner. Diane was 51, divorced for two years and not searching for another committed relationship—though not opposed to meeting a nice guy.

Stu turned out to be 17 years older, which Diane deemed too steep a difference. Her husband of 20-plus years had been almost a decade older, and she had decided a man her age would be a better fit.

Still, she liked Stu well enough. When he walked her out to her car after dinner, she noticed how comfortable he seemed in his body, how relaxed and at ease his movements were.

Stu was a seasonal visitor to Diane's city, and over the next six weeks they went out sporadically. When he returned to town the next year, they did the same, though Diane was dating someone else by then. Nevertheless, she and Stu continued their friendship.

The third year he came to town, Diane wasn't dating anyone steadily and neither was Stu. Their time together became more frequent, but was never physical.

Then one night, after a movie, dinner and a walk on the beach, they climbed back into Stu's car for the drive home, still talking and laughing, when suddenly Stu leaned over and kissed

Diane. She was only a little surprised; she'd been wondering exactly what she'd do if Stu tried to take things in this direction. She wasn't at all convinced she wanted a new lover.

But everything felt so right. She liked the pressure of Stu's lips, the feel of his hands cupping her face, the way he pulled slightly away and then delved back to kiss her deeply. A minute later Stu broke the kiss, saying, "My heart is pounding so hard."

"Mine too," she said, and pulled him back for another.

Five minutes of exquisite kissing later, all Diane could think about was how much she wanted to be in bed with Stu. If he was this great at kissing, how great might he be at everything else, she wondered.

Nevertheless, Diane says she began mentally forming a list of why a sexual relationship with someone new was a bad idea. What about her reputation? What would her mother say? Was it really a good idea to get involved sexually?

She was up to item five before she realized the list belonged to a teenager, not a grown woman, and none of her automatic roadblocks applied any longer.

At that point, she says she totally gave in to the make-out session.

Stu's convertible wasn't roomy, however, and sometime later she declared, "Okay. This is as turned on as I'm willing to get in the front seat of your car. We've got to figure something out."

Neither one had a place to themselves that night, so they made a date for the next weekend, content to let the delicious passion simmer. Those first kisses turned out to be an accurate barometer for everything that followed, and the pair became a couple. Though separated by distance, they find ways to be together every month or so for marathon kissing and lovemaking sessions.

As Diane says, "I waited all my life for a guy who kisses like this. Who cares how old he is?"

In Dulce's case, the power of kissing led to her marriage, now a lusty, 32-year union. In fact, the 50-year-old Latino mother of two gleefully shared stories from one of the most active sex lives of anyone interviewed for this book.

"I like to be kissed. I want to be kissed all the time," she confesses. "But men should not go into the kissing too soon. They should be able to sense when she's ready. Kissing is almost like having sex."

Dulce knew her future husband, Freddy, for six months before they kissed, and says if he had pushed physical contact earlier, she would have rejected him.

"I was a little afraid of his age," she says. She was just 18 when she met Freddy, a Dominican man, at her girlfriend's wedding. "He was a man and I was a little girl. My mother didn't know he was 27. He looked young."

Though Dulce's first instinct was to run, she took the time to get to know Freddy, and says she started to see his softer side after about a month.

"And that smile. And those lips," she says. "At some point I told him I was finishing high school, and that's when he knew how old I was."

They dated for six months, but Dulce wouldn't kiss him. Though she'd kissed other boys, she was a virgin and wary of Freddy's obvious experience.

But then came the serenade.

"We were at my house," Dulce recalls. "He took out his guitar and started singing to me. He sang these beautiful love songs in Spanish. He sings so beautiful."

He strolled outside to continue the serenade, which Dulce

says sent her mother—and others—into a state of high amusement.

"I lived in an Italian neighborhood, and all these old Italians were out there listening and watching. I was blushing. I was red in the face. I was telling him to get inside. But he wanted to get that [passionate] action in me, you know?"

And he did. That evening, when Freddy eventually put his guitar aside, the couple found themselves alone in the family room, with Dulce perched a bit warily on their 1970s-era sofa, a round sectional with open ends.

"He kept getting closer; I knew sooner or later we had to kiss," Dulce says. "So I kept moving, playing hard to get. My heart was beating like a hundred miles an hour. And I was getting all hot and bothered big-time. It was bad. I thought, 'What happens when he kisses me and I don't like it? I've been leading him on for six months, so what will I tell him?'

"I'm all flustered and he's getting closer. He looks at me with those deep, dark eyes and those luscious lips and he gets close to me and he holds my hands and he says, 'You know I love you.'

"It wasn't a peck; it was a luscious kiss. He grabbed the bottom lip and kissed me so thoroughly I heard bells in my head and ringing in my ears. I felt like my head was all full of air and I couldn't even think. I was so close to the edge of the sofa that I just slid right off of it onto the floor!

"The word that came out of my mouth was, 'Wow.' I was stunned.

"He was worried. He picked me up and put me back and asked if I was okay. And I said, 'Can we try that again?'

"And we did. We must have kissed for 45 minutes nonstop. Every kiss was passionate, and every part of me wanted to be with him. I didn't feel scared anymore. I felt completely like I could trust him and that whatever he did wouldn't be bad.

"It was very, very romantic. I will never forget it."

Three months later, the couple married. Dulce said she knew the magic she felt when they kissed would pave the way for whatever lay ahead.

"Most of the wedding pictures were of us kissing," says Dulce. "It's all we wanted to do. The photographer said he'd never seen such a happy bride and groom. We had to hide from him so we could kiss. He was following us, but we wanted to be alone already. It was time. We ran away from the reception while everyone was still dancing.

"When we got to the apartment, I was getting nervous. I thought, 'How am I going to please this man? When we kiss it's so beautiful, but how will I please him?'

"We opened all the gifts and drank some champagne. And then I went and changed. Finally, we're lying in bed and he's kissing me. He kissed my neck and my arms. He knew he could calm me down that way. The kissing was the bridge. My favorite is he kissed my ankles. After that, forget about it! I was lost. Inside I was already lost in my passion.

"He kissed the inside of my thighs and worked up to my lips again. There was so much fire in my body. When I was naked I felt beautiful. He was very gentle with me and didn't hurt me at all. I bet we lasted two hours. It was just total ecstasy for me."

True to its auspicious beginning, Dulce said the sex life she's built with her fiery lover is completely satisfying, and the couple still enjoys sex daily.

"I think our sex life got better," she says. "We started discovering new things. I would discover something I liked and say, 'Do it this way.' And he'd say, 'Can you try this, this way?'

"We got a book that had all the positions, and every night

we'd say, 'Let's try this one.' It was fun. When you're young you want to learn new things. It's about pleasing not one, but both of you. We tried everything once, some only twice, and some we kept in the routine because they were very, very good."

In Dulce's words, sex "keeps us out of stress.

"I want sex every night," she admits. "Even when we get upset with each other—and believe me, we've had fights—one of us always makes up. If we have the energy for two times, we go two rounds. Morning sex is the best. But every night, yes, we do. We have some kind of sex. It doesn't have to be penetration every time. Oral sex is wonderful. I would never say no to oral sex."

Her children are now 29 and 27, but when they were teens, they would occasionally question their mom as to whether they were planned or surprises.

"Whenever the kids ask if they're 'oops,' I say no," Dulce laughs. "I tell them, 'You guys are here because your dad is a good kisser.'"

FURTHER ADVENTURES IN KISSING

Though kissing never led to children for Judy, the thrice-married, now single 51-year-old shares one trait with the two previous women: She decided to have sex with a guy based on his fine kissing skills. But it took her almost four decades to get there.

She kissed Mike for the first time when she was 12, says Judy, a voluptuous, long-haired brunette.

"Between 12 and 16 we were doing a lot of necking—no petting, just necking. He was a good boy. He didn't even know I knew he got a hard-on, but girls know these things."

Her memories of those innocent times are vivid all these

years later. She clearly remembers when they both had leads in the school play, *Flowers for Algernon*.

"We were waiting backstage for our parts and the stage had big, black velvet curtains," she says. "He came over to me and gave me this look, and I spun the curtains around us and we kissed. The audience had no idea."

Though their relationship ended after high school ("We were just teenagers hot for each other"), the memory of Mike's kisses stayed with Judy through three marriages. In 2002, the high school sweethearts reconnected online.

He was all the way across the country, but it was a sure thing that they'd figure out a way to bridge the distance. Mike was divorced; Judy was still married, but had decided to end it six months earlier and was saving money to be independent. Mike used a visit to his aunt as a pretext and arrived in Judy's hometown a month later.

"When he got off the plane and leaned in to kiss my cheek, I felt like I was 12 years old again. We exchanged pecks on the cheek, and as we separated, our cheeks brushed and I could smell his essence."

His smell proved irresistible, and so instead of stepping back completely, Judy kissed his lips.

After all that time, was Mike still a good kisser?

"Yes! It was a passionate, exploratory kiss," she says. "It was wonderful. Memorable. We were in the airport parking lot, standing in the pathway of passengers. We had to have been there 20 minutes! Somebody came by twice [coming and going] and said, 'You're still here!' We'd been necking the whole time."

Despite the passionate greeting, Judy said she and Mike "played good all weekend," behaving decorously around family, friends and even Judy's husband. They socialized at gatherings and enjoyed their simmering passion.

On his last day in town, Mike stopped by Judy's place to say good-bye.

"I stayed home from work to make him breakfast," recalls Judy. "My husband had gone to work, and I let Mike in. I kissed him immediately; I grabbed his shirt collar and said, 'I'm going to know you'—'know' in the biblical sense. We didn't make it to the guest bedroom. We only got as far as the living room floor."

Gone were Mike's teenage reservations; Judy says he didn't hesitate.

"He went right for it. Face in the crotch right now. I never came so fast in my life," she says. "I never released myself to anyone that fast."

Though their torrid lovemaking was as good as she'd hoped for all those years, Judy and Mike are an on-again, off-again couple. In the years since they reconnected, Judy has tried to break things off twice, unsuccessfully.

"I've loved him all my life," she says, "but on a day-to-day basis, I wonder if I can live with him, live with his criticisms. He thinks I should be ashamed of my marriages and my past. And I'm just not."

Even so, she does enjoy their physical connection—kisses and all.

IN THE ABSENCE OF KISSING

While such stories demonstrate the passionate power of kissing, tales of marriages that have morphed into practically sexless unions always seem to outnumber them.

"Women complain of low desire on a daily basis in my practice," says Dr. Whelihan. Studies show 43 percent of women have sexual complaints, but in Mo's practice, where her clients know it's more than okay to discuss sex, almost 90 percent of her patients between the ages of 40 and 55 complain of low desire. There are good reasons for this. These are the years in a woman's life when she's raising teenagers, with their complicated problems; juggling a full-time job that's heavy with responsibility; struggling to keep a decades-old marriage fresh; maintaining friendships; running a household; and perhaps caring for her own or her spouse's aging parents. Energy for sex is hard to come by.

So how to inflame desire? Since our survey shows kissing as a key ingredient for stimulating desire, it would seem reasonable to presume it's a good starting point for couples. And yet, during her speaking engagements—whether she's addressing her fellow physicians or a community club—when Dr. Whelihan asks married men or women to think back to the last time they engaged in just making out . . . they can't seem to remember! Somewhere in the day-in, day-out routine of long-term marriages, sensual kissing gets relegated to the "irrelevant" list.

Accumulated emotional baggage is surely part of the problem. The small aggravations of daily life (he never remembers to take out the trash; he always leaves his dirty clothes on the floor) add up to major resentments. And the sheer proximity of a partner encourages us to take him or her for granted, reasoning that our partner's lips and body will always be available to us.

But it's a mistake to dismiss kissing as insignificant. Think back for a moment to your first truly romantic encounter. Remember the shiver of anticipation you had for your lover's kiss, the melting together you once felt when your lips met? The seduction of a passionate kiss is so overwhelming that women throughout history have admitted to throwing their chaste intentions to the wind and allowing their desire to lead them to bed after all.

As divorcée Mia insists, "Kissing can be just as arousing if not more so than any other kind of foreplay."

IT'S IN HIS KISS

What's so great about a kiss? Why do women report that they love to watch the sexy, passionate kissing scenes in movies and that it stimulates their own desire?

Dr. Helen Fischer, an anthropologist at Rutgers University who has studied mating behaviors for 30 years and made numerous television appearances, says the testosterone levels found in male saliva are passed to the woman during a passionate kiss, thereby increasing her testosterone and sexy thoughts. Fischer says a sexy kiss also raises levels of dopamine, a chemical in the brain that makes women crave their partner.

Dr. Whelihan adds that men may want to keep in mind that dancing, sexy music and touch also initiate a dopamine surge, thereby stimulating sexual desire.

Clearly, kissing deserves a starring role in a couple's lovemaking repertoire. But what constitutes a sexy kiss?

It's different for everyone, which is why lovers are so elated to find a compatible partner. Nevertheless, based on our survey, there seem to be some common denominators. Women who aren't big fans of kissing most often cited "too wet" as the reason. "My guy is like a Saint Bernard; he drools too much!" says one woman. Several older survey respondents said they found a partner's tongue in their mouth "disgusting."

Nevertheless, plenty of women answer "a wet kiss" when asked what stimulates their desire.

Some recommendations for a good kiss from our survey respondents are that it should not cover the whole mouth at once or suck all the air out or be too forceful. Soft lips and good oral hygiene are key components.

Also mentioned is the heightened sexual anticipation that accompanies small nibbles around the mouth and gentle sucking on the lips.

"Kissing relays a message of wanting," says Dr. Whelihan. "I challenge you to spend two minutes of passionate kissing daily. I guarantee it will markedly increase your partner's sexual interest."

Boyfriends? Lovers? Husbands? Anyone listening?

DECADES OF DESIRE:
THE TEENS

"I don't like it when a guy won't go down on me; it's a deal-breaker," says Sasha, 21. "I broke up with a guy who wouldn't go down on me. That's what I love."

"I prop my head up on a pillow so I can watch him [performing oral sex] or us making love because that helps me reach orgasm," says Hailey, 19. "I've tried earplugs too, so I can concentrate on what's going on. And I'm kind of into toys; I bring those into bed. I know he's not going to last, so I'll masturbate while we have intercourse; whatever gets you there."

"I'm learning something new all the time," says Soha, 20, a college junior who is still in a relationship with her first partner after more than two years. "I love sex; I want it all the time." Her quickest route to orgasm, she says, is "cowgirl"—on top—or from behind, with vaginal entry. "His hands on my hips . . . I love that, 'cause you both have control. And we can both reach my clitoris. He can reach around or I can put my finger there and it's just better with both at the same time."

These are not the words of shy, shrinking violets. In fact, it doesn't seem a stretch to award the label "empowered" to the teens we interviewed about sexual desire.

Since the youngest person to complete our survey on sexual desire was 15, the teen "decade" is actually half a decade. A total of 27 women 19 or younger took the survey, and though some had turned 20 or 21 when interviewed for this chapter, we allowed them to remain classified as teens. The lapse between the time they took our survey and their interview enables them to speak to the entire experience of sexual desire in their teen years, and how it evolved throughout that decade.

As a group, the teens are unself-conscious, unabashed and comfortable speaking about all aspects of sex. Admittedly, Dr. Whelihan's most reticent or shy patients may have chosen not to fill out a survey in her office, so it's possible our sampling is weighted toward confident extroverts.

Nevertheless, the responses from teens indicate that their hormones are hyperactive, and their desire is stimulated most notably by scent and their partner's manliness, but also by breast stimulation and kissing around the ears and neck. During sex, many say, they are thinking about what they can do to make things better, more fun or spicier. Some wonder what is going on in their partner's brain, and a few wonder if they're "doing it right."

Among the eight women in this age group interviewed in depth, no particular age emerged as the average for when they first had intercourse. Every age—from 13 to 19—was claimed, with 15 being the only age mentioned twice.

The teens' level of experience was likewise varied: Several had only a single lover; one said her total was around 20; another said it was more than 40. The rest had a single-digit number.

But there were similarities. The majority of the young women were quick to bring up their preference for assertive, manly, in-charge partners in the bedroom, and all but one gave indications of an already-empowered sense of sexuality.

In fact, the teens we met were generally well-informed and ready to collect on their expectation of satisfying sex.

Consider Daisy, now 20, who estimates she's been with 20 lovers. She became sexually active the day after her 14th birthday, and shares that since it takes her a long time to orgasm, she teases her lovers to prolong the process.

"I'll switch positions, or if I'm giving oral sex, I'll go slow. If I feel them start to tense up, I'll tease them in another way."

Her results are impressive: "I have orgasms about 90 percent of the time," she says, "and that's not true of my other girlfriends," who sometimes tell her they "don't get how to do it."

Daisy says she's been fortunate to date older guys, which she feels helps. Plus, she knows what she likes.

"I don't feel uncomfortable having sex. I know what I'm doing and know how to push them to the edge."

Even less experienced Allison, 21, who's with her third sexual partner, displays evidence of sexual empowerment. When she met her current boyfriend, she says he "didn't give oral sex at all."

How did she change his mind?

Simple. "I stopped giving him head."

HORMONES vs. HEARSAY

During the interview process, a somewhat curious commonality was observed in this age group: Not one young woman mentioned good old-fashioned horniness as a factor in her decision to have sex the first time. Instead, a combination of curiosity, peer pressure and a desire to be closer to their boyfriends guided the choice. The natural urgings of their physical bodies were precluded or perhaps drowned out by messages from friends, media and society, all urging them to jump-start their sexuality.

"I didn't want to go into high school as a virgin," says Daisy. "The majority of my friends at the time were seniors or graduated. I wanted to feel more comfortable with myself, more confident. When talking about sexuality with my friends, I wanted to relate and be more comfortable around those discussions."

Samantha, whose first experience was at 15, believed her friends when they said sex would bring her closer to her boyfriend.

"It actually did intensify my emotions for him, but not his for me," she says now, at 21. "It fell apart after that. I was getting so clingy because I did have sex with him."

In subsequent romantic encounters, Samantha retained the belief that sex would strengthen the bond. "I think I felt insecure in the relationships," she says, "like, 'I need to do this because I want to be a good girlfriend.'"

Allison, who capitulated to her boyfriend just a few days before her 16th birthday, said timing was the deciding factor.

"I kind of liked being a virgin, being innocent, but I had been dating him six or seven months, so that was it. I had done everything else, so I thought, 'Big deal, what the heck.'"

The couple was on a cruise with Allison's parents and found they could escape to his locked stateroom for privacy.

"The last thing you want is to be interrupted the first time," she quips.

Allison acknowledges that there were also physical reasons she wanted to have sex, but doesn't directly reference her own desire. Instead, she notes that others had made it "sound fun."

But her first time "wasn't great" she recalls. "It was okay. . . . I was on my period, so there was lots of lubrication, and that was good."

Hailey's first time happened with her boyfriend of one year, well into her 15th year.

"I'm a woodsy girl, and we were out in the woods on a four-wheeler. We were kissing and it just went on from there. We knew no one could see us. We got touchy-feely; I was definitely ready at that point."

She indicates that she was tired of thinking about it, of not knowing.

"I was always scared—of the pain, of getting pregnant, of my mom finding out, would people be able to tell, am I going to be different, will I turn into a whore?"

Does she have any regrets?

"Kind of, because it was my virginity and because it was really bad," she says. "It lasted only about two seconds. He was only good at kissing, nothing else. But that was all I knew. When I think back on it now, I realize that it was not good at all."

A simple desire for sex is also missing from Annabelle's explanation for why she chose her first lover, though she waited longer than others.

"I initiated it. I was just ready to have a partner. I was 19 and couldn't take it anymore," she shares. Annabelle broke off the relationship after a year and a half: "He was a horrible person all around. I don't know why I picked him. He did this thing when I was naked . . . he'd point out all my flaws. It made me so self-conscious."

She has yet to take another lover.

Sasha got started much younger, at 13. "I said yes to my friend's brother; he was 17," she says. "It was kind of like impressing him. I had big boobs since I was little, and always loved older guys. He said, 'You've done this before, right?' I said yes; I played it cool. But I went to cry somewhere later, alone."

Why the tears?

"He was Brazilian and he was huge," she shares.

Hayden, who had sex the first time shortly after she turned 17, says she doesn't regret the "when" of her first time, but she does regret the "how."

"I said I wouldn't do it without it being romantic," she recalls. "I wanted candles and flowers and all that stuff my first time. It ended up being the complete opposite; we were just crazy one night after drinking. I just gave in because I knew I'd been wanting to. It was the right time but not the right circumstances."

Hayden, who's now 18 and still with her partner, wryly notes that she wanted flowers for her prom too, but her boyfriend got her liquor.

"He's the ultimate man's man," she explains. "He's not a sensitive guy whatsoever. I'm the complete opposite."

Soha is a bit of an exception. Raised by a single mom in an economically depressed farming community, she's now a college junior at 20. Soha gave considerable thought to her decision to have sex, which she eventually did at 18. Demonstrating exceptional maturity, she says she learned from her friends' mistakes.

"I had friends doing it for all the wrong reasons. I knew that [even] when I was a freshman in high school," she recalls. "People were saying, 'You should do it; you don't know what you're missing.' My response was, 'You can't miss what you haven't had.' Or I'd say, 'Nah, I've waited this long; I can wait a little longer.'

"What they would actually say was, 'You need some dick in your life,'" she confides with a laugh. "But some of the girls who were saying that, I felt were promiscuous. I was like, 'No, thank you.'

"A lot of girls like me [raised by a single mom] were looking for a male figure to love them, and I wasn't really interested in that. My mom was enough. I'm an only child and I get a lot of attention. Mom always told me I was pretty and beautiful, so I wasn't susceptible to thinking I liked a guy just because he said I was beautiful. It was just a nice compliment."

Soha believes 14 or 15 is too soon to have sex.

"You don't know what you're doing. You don't know if you truly love a person . . . well, maybe you do, but you have to make sure you're really ready, and aroused—or is he the horny one trying to talk you into it? And why are you doing it? Is it because *you* love him or you want *him* to love you? And how are you going to feel about it the next day? Are you still going to respect yourself? And in a worst-case scenario, if there's a breakup, how will you feel?

"I answered all those questions before I had sex with my boyfriend," she explains. "We were exclusive for eight months before we had sex. I'm surprised I had sex with him. I thought that was kind of soon, but I really was ready. I always said I was going to wait two years before I gave up anything."

So how did he change her mind?

He didn't.

"I changed my mind," she says. "He was a good guy. He never pressured me. All guys will say, 'I love you . . . whenever you're ready.' But he meant it. He never said, 'I love you; I think it's time.' A couple of times I said, 'Let's do it,' and he said, 'Are you sure you want this? No, you're not.'"

Soha came to realize that even if they eventually broke up, she'd be okay with her decision, because, "I'm not doing it because I want him to love me; I'm doing it because we love each other and it's a deeper expression of love.

"I never felt that [sex] was all he was there for. I was like,

'I truly love this person, and even if it doesn't last forever, I'm really okay with this guy having that part of me.' My first time was a good experience. It was slow; it was gentle; it was loving."

ORGASMS: EASY OR ELUSIVE?

Like most gynecologists, Dr. Whelihan has seen abundant evidence of the trend toward early sexual behavior.

"In general, girls I see in my practice today are not influenced by the cultural/moral issues and don't think it is a big deal if they have sex," she says. "Not only is the age of sexual activity getting younger, there's been a shift in how young girls view their sexuality. These days, girls are just as curious as boys about sex and not bashful about exploring."

As she inquires about sexual activity on the part of her patients, Dr. Whelihan finds many girls in middle school have given oral sex to boys, and some have received as well.

"They don't seem bashful in telling me these things, which I find a little surprising. Maybe since I don't criticize and am not a figure of authority, they know I'll accept the answer they give me.

"Girls understand the power of giving oral sex to a boy from a very young age," Dr. Mo continues, "and the boys—although awkward—are going along for the exciting ride. Girls often seem to be the initiators."

Girls as young as 12 and 13 in Dr. Mo's practice are having intercourse, she says, but it's more common at 15 and after.

"The youngest ones are mostly having sex with boys 16 to 18, and they don't seem worried that sex with guys older than 18 is illegal. I'm not condoning this, and their comments are just hearsay. My duty is to educate the girls about the risks and make sure they are not being coerced."

Many of the 15-year-old girls "brag" to their doctor that they were the experienced ones in their encounter and the boy was the virgin. Dr. Whelihan speculates that the general empowerment of girls in our society, with females receiving more equal treatment in sports and education, is now trickling into the arena of sexuality.

But despite the presence of entitled, early-adopter teens, young women still struggle with an array of sexual issues.

Hayden, the young woman who began having sex with her boyfriend shortly after her 17th birthday, has yet to experience an orgasm though they've been together a year.

"I've done it a number of times; I thought I'd have one," she says, wondering aloud whether she's doing something wrong. "I have other friends who almost always have orgasms."

Maybe they do . . . and maybe they don't.

Certainly several of the teens interviewed here were highly successful in that arena, but it's worth noting that for this age group—and 20-somethings as well—a frequent answer to the question, "What's the biggest lie you were told about sex?" centers around the misconception that each and every sexual experience will be special, memorable, ecstatic and—by extension—orgasmic.

"People make it seem that women have an orgasm all of the time, which is not true and, in fact, is very difficult for some of us," writes one 18-year-old survey respondent.

A 21-year-old answers the "biggest lie" question with, "That you get off every time. I sure as hell don't!" And a 20-year-old agrees, saying the biggest lie is that you orgasm every time, or else she "hasn't met the right person" to have that experience.

This expectation that orgasms will occur with every sexual encounter isn't passed down from the older generation. Very few mature women discussing sex with a curious, inexperienced girl would lead her to expect 100 percent success. So it is today's younger generation—with an assist from popular media—that is passing this particular falsehood around among themselves: i.e., sisters, boyfriends, boasting girlfriends.

(In contrast with the teens and twenties, it's worth noting that the "biggest lies" middle-aged women recall are mostly fabrications created by their elders to stop them from having sex, such as "if you kiss a boy in the dark you'll get pregnant." Whereas misinformation once came from cautious adults, now it comes from peers.)

Sasha, the woman who lost her virginity to the Brazilian, says that with "regular sex" she has orgasms maybe 30 percent of the time. With masturbation or oral sex, it's much higher, more like 90 percent.

Samantha, who experienced her first orgasm through masturbation at age 13, was 19 when she had her first orgasm from oral sex. Now 21, she has yet to experience orgasm with penetration from any of her eight partners.

Allison says that if her current boyfriend performs oral sex, she has orgasms 99 percent of the time; with intercourse it's more like 10 percent.

Hailey has orgasms 80 percent of the time with intercourse, but notes that she brings toys to bed, knowing they generally ensure success.

Then there's the previously mentioned Daisy (90 percent) and Soha, the latter of whom says she orgasms during 85 percent of sexual encounters with her boyfriend.

Survey-wide, it's interesting to note that only about 15 percent of teens say oral sex is their quickest route to orgasm, which is the smallest percentage of any decade until the eighties. By comparison, almost 26 percent of women in their thirties, 19 percent of women in their fifties and 21 percent of 60-something women name oral sex as their quickest route to orgasm.

However, the survey shows that there are women of all ages who have yet to experience an orgasm, so teenagers led to believe it magically occurs with all sexual encounters—even loving ones—are being fed a fantasy by their contemporaries.

BE A MAN!

Sensitive, caring boyfriends are fine with teenage girls, but *not* in the bedroom. Again and again, women this age verbalize the desire for a powerful, assertive sex partner.

"I like it when men are kind of aggressive and dominant," says Samantha. "He doesn't have to be manly in every pursuit, but I want him dominant in that way. I like confidence, not cockiness. If he's like, 'I can get any girl,' that's not appealing. So he can be quiet and sweet every other place, but in the bedroom, that would be what I like."

Samantha enjoys sex with her current boyfriend, but does wish he'd be more aggressive. Nonetheless, she definitely doesn't like dirty talk in the bedroom. (Her example: "You like my dick in your pussy?") "It makes me feel dirty and I get turned off," she says of comments like this.

(Since other survey respondents of all ages mentioned dirty talk as something that specifically stimulates their desire, men would do well to ask their partner what turns her on. And women should readily share what variety of whisperings they enjoy—or prepare to be disappointed.)

Hailey, 19, is a freshman in college who's had seven lovers. Like many other teens, she prefers a dominant sexual partner.

"I'm attracted to bigger men, calluses on their hands, workingmen. I like tough boys, not the scrawny ones in the corner filing their nails and wearing Abercrombie. I love rough sex. . . . I like him in control, totally. Don't *ask* me to do something: tell me what you want or put me there. I like to be thrown around . . . to know they want you that bad."

A partner who stays totally silent turns Hailey off. She doesn't need a running commentary, but expects to hear that he's having a good time, that he's enjoying what they're doing. Otherwise, she wonders, "Am I not pleasuring you?"

When reminiscing about her only lover, Annabelle echoes some of these sentiments.

"I sometimes liked slow sex, but not usually. My 'primitive' Annabelle really wanted to rip his clothes off. I wanted it rough sometimes. When I would take his shirt off, I would want to throw it off, but he'd want to make sure it didn't get wrinkled. It was so annoying. All his clothes had to be on a chair: they couldn't touch the floor. I hated that. I wanted him to be more aggressive; I wanted him to rip my clothes off. He was too much like a girly girl for me."

Daisy too: "I'm a farm girl, so I like rough hands. I'm old-fashioned. I like a guy who's very in control, wanting it his way and me wanting to please him no matter what."

She says her quickest route to orgasm is, "him talking dirty, being very possessive, the whole masculinity about it." She likes cowgirl style, "with him gripping me."

It seems logical that less experienced teens would respond to strong, take-charge partners, since that type of lover would allay any feelings of insecurity a novice might harbor. But Dr. Whelihan notes that women of all ages find themselves attracted to the rough-hewn bad boy.

"Perhaps it is because they are a bit more aggressive, which may be due to a higher testosterone level," she says. "Perhaps we are attracted to that pheromone. Women often describe liking their partner better when he 'takes what he wants' or 'puts me where he wants me.' And all women, particularly married ones, say they are truly turned off by the whining man who begs for sex.

"It seems as much as we women like to tell men what to do in every other aspect of life, when it comes to sex, we like the confident, slightly aggressive guy who knows what he wants."

LESS BUTT, PLEASE

Not surprisingly, almost 60 percent of the teenagers surveyed (27, if you remember) say they're still waiting for the best sex of their lives.

During sex, they tend to stay in the moment and are able to block out everyday distractions, an ability that often decreases as women become more sexually experienced. Thirty-three percent of teens say pleasing their partner and thinking of how to enhance the sex they're having is what's in their head during sex. Just 18.5 percent of women in their twenties say they stay fully present in the moment during sex, and only 9 percent of women in their thirties.

When asked for one thing they wish their partners would not do in regard to sex, 44 percent of teens have no complaints. "Nothing. He's great," is a common answer. Rushing to intercourse did come up, but only one teen answered "anal sex" on the survey.

That seemed too low to us, considering that almost 12 percent of women survey-wide said requests for anal sex was their premier complaint. So when we interviewed the teens group, we asked the young women about it specifically. When we did, this decade actually ended up having the highest percent-age—18.2—of women who said this was the one thing they wish their partner would *not* do.

All the teens say they field frequent, ongoing appeals for this variation.

"I'm up to try anything once," says Daisy. "But I don't want him to try to force anal."

How, specifically, does she deal with direct attempts?

"I squirm to avoid anal; I try to play it off," she says, "like, 'I don't know what you're talking about.' I've had it pretty often, but it's still not one of my favorite things. I'll do it for him, but I don't get the whole point.

"Guys do ask for it right away," she affirms. "It's one of those things, if you're just getting to know someone, you'll share what you like and don't."

She and former lovers have "discussed" such topics via phone.

"People are more comfortable texting than talking," she says of the practice. "[You avoid] having someone laugh at your question and answer."

Helpfully, Daisy explains how anal sex has assumed a larger importance for today's teens than previous generations. There's a hierarchy, it seems.

"It's like, yeah, you've had sex, and you've done oral sex—now it's a whole new chapter to have anal sex. It's a whole different step."

She's not a fan.

"I'm talkative and open, but for me, [anal sex] doesn't get me where I want to be. Only occasionally will I do that, [because] it pleases me to please him. If I'm with a person I'm not going to date, and it's just a hookup, I wouldn't do anal sex. If it's someone

I'm with and have a relationship with, then it's part of building a connection, understanding each other better emotionally and physically. But I never think, 'I really desire anal sex.'"

"I will not engage in anal sex," says Soha, who is still with her original lover. "My boyfriend hasn't ever asked for it. I considered it once and brought it up to him, but he said if a guy would do it to a girl, then he'd do it to a boy. I won't do it mainly for health reasons; I heard it's not good for you."

"I've always found it painful," says Allison, who's tried it with all three of her partners. "I don't ever ask for it. If they want to, I try it, but I usually end up pissed off, because it hurts. I'm like, 'Fuck you.' It bothers me that they want to try it, even knowing that it will hurt me."

"I do not like anal sex," echoes Sasha, who waited six years after becoming sexually active to try it the first time. The occasion was her 19th birthday, and she notes that she was drunk and doesn't remember much.

Of her 40 partners, Sasha estimates that maybe 10 have asked her to try anal sex. "After a couple of times [having sex], they're ready to ask," she affirms. On occasion, she's been brutally blunt with those doing the asking.

"I've definitely said to them, 'If you want to stick your dick in someone's ass, go find a guy, 'cause I've got something else that works.' Or, 'Let me stick something up *your* ass.'"

Though Sasha mentions a girl in her high school who let it be known that she'd "rather have it up the ass because she said it's easier for her to get off," Sasha isn't inclined in that direction.

"I can't relax," she says. "I actually tried it drunk two nights ago; it was just my second time."

Because her boyfriend of two months, whom she loves, was asking, she was willing to try again, but "I tensed up and it hurt so bad. I don't think I'd try it again."

Hailey has had more success with anal sex than her fellow teens. She's tried it only with her current boyfriend of two years (who is her seventh partner).

"I've had orgasms that way, but it was because the clitoris was stimulated too," she says. "I don't really like it. We've probably tried it 10 times. I've stopped a few times, but three times we kept going. It hurts really bad; I have to distract myself. If I have a toy I can focus on that pleasure instead; they kind of go together and that can be better. If I had to choose, I'd say, 'No, I don't want to do that again.' But after you get used to it, it's all right. But I don't like the feeling. You feel constipated."

Annabelle falls into the same camp.

"I've been told it's really uncomfortable and it feels like you have to poop the whole time and it hurts," she said.

Her only lover would often ask about it, saying someone at his job told him it was "really fun" and they should try it. Annabelle declined.

"I feel like men who want to try that are curious about their own sexuality," she says. "I don't want to try anal at all. It seems much more painful than enjoyable. I said [to my boyfriend], 'Let me do a strap-on,' and he didn't want to do that. See, they don't want it done to them, but they want to do it to you. Maybe it is a dominant thing. Or when they want to humiliate you."

EVOLVING DESIRE

I wrap up the interviews with the teenagers by asking the young women to consider the evolution of their sexual desire throughout their teen years. What changes in themselves and in their sexual desire did they notice from the time they became sexually active—whether 13 or 19—until now? And how do they see their desire evolving in the future?

Quiet 18-year-old Hayden hopes her active libido doesn't diminish.

"When I get older, I don't know if my sexual desire will go down, even though right now I feel like I'm ready all the time. I wake up and think about it; around the house I think about it; at night I think, 'Oh, my God, I wanna do it.' When I hear people talk about sex being boring, I just hope I never get like that, like there's no time [for sex] and it's not the same. I want to never be like that. I want my husband to still look at me that way."

Daisy, the self-described farm girl, says that when she's dating someone, she wants sex all the time.

"It's more of a desire and a need now," she explains. "Before it was more of a want and, 'hmm, something fun.' At 20, I want it more than I did at, say, 16. If I'm dating someone, I constantly want sexual interaction, whether it's fooling around or going all the way. If it's a hookup, and it's more than one time, I feel like I want it with them constantly. I'm like a guy in that I'm not so tensed up and stressed if I can have sex more often. It's something relaxing; it can reach me on another level and make me feel like everything's all right."

Sasha, who at 21 has eight years of experience, finds her new love of two months has brought a big shift in her sexual desire.

"Now romance has to be involved," she says. "Now that I know what it's like to have sex with somebody I love, I don't want to have sex without that. He looks into my eyes when we're making love. That's huge. I never had that before. It's so deep, like he's looking into my soul. When I love somebody, [the sex] is good every time, even if I don't orgasm.

"I used to want it more often. I was a party girl, so it was kind of fun for me. If I wanted to have sex it was just going to happen. Now I'm thinking about our relationship and settling down. Now that I've had the good sex with him, I'm like, why did I waste my time?"

And though she once talked openly with her girlfriends about sex, Sasha says with this new boyfriend, it's different. She doesn't want another woman poaching her lover.

"I haven't told any stories. I don't want other people knowing what I have."

Allison, on the other hand, hasn't noticed any shifts in her sexuality since she became active around her 16th birthday.

"My desire hasn't really changed except that I want it more if I've just had it. If [the sex you're having] is really good, you want it more. If it's just okay, you forget how good it can be. You lose desire if you don't have orgasms. It's like, why not just go to sleep?"

Samantha, now 21 with six years' experience, says her sexual drive has experienced some ups and downs.

"Back in the day, when I was 15, it was based largely on curiosity, as well as wanting to be emotionally closer and strengthening the relationship with my boyfriend. We broke up, but got back together several times [over a period of four years]. I would date guys in between, but I would be having sex with some of them because I think it made me feel powerful and desired. That's what fueled it. I'd brag to friends about how I couldn't live without sex.

"But as I got into college, after my boyfriend and I broke up for good, my desire died down. I waited about a year and didn't have a partner. I guess I was in a fallow period."

With her current boyfriend, Samantha doesn't think about sex as often as she used to.

"Now it's a lot more controlled; I'm a lot busier; I'm going to be a teacher and I intern with young girls. Still, when I start my period, oh, my God, I get this urge where I really want to have sex *now*. Otherwise, I just want to go to sleep."

Samantha, like Sasha, no longer talks with girlfriends about sex like she once did.

"Back then, I'd tell 'this is what I did' stories and we'd all laugh, but maybe we don't want to laugh about it anymore," she says. "I think I'm ashamed of my past, just the number of sexual partners I've had [eight], and feeling like that's not cool. Back then, I would sleep with a guy I wasn't boyfriend/girlfriend with. Now I've settled down and am just with him [her current boyfriend]. I like him a lot. Now I feel I'm not just hooking up with random guys."

Soha, the teen who was slow to make her decision, says her sexual desire is stronger now than when she became active at 18.

"I want him more," she admits. "I think I'm still getting closer to him as time goes on. As we get closer and older, I'm being drawn more to him and my desire is increasing. And sex makes you think about babies, and I think, 'Oh, my God, I want to have kids with him someday.' And he's the same way."

Hailey, who's had three years' experience and seven lovers, says her sex life has "definitely gotten better, because I've learned new things and had sex with several partners. I've had different experiences, not the same thing over and over. I've had good and I've had bad, so I'm not as willing to put up with bad sex. Now, if it's not good, I crave something new. I don't want the same thing over and over."

Annabelle says one big change for her is that she's not as trusting now as when she was 19.

"Things would have been a lot different if I'd had a different first partner who was more accepting of my body," says the tall, beautifully shaped young woman. "I would have had more fun too. I don't think I'm as naive now. Before I wanted it to be one person forever, and I know now men aren't like that. If a guy wanted an open relationship, I'd be more open to that now. Although I would prefer a monogamous relationship, I know it doesn't always work out like that."

Annabelle's learned she "just can't deal with people putting me down. Words are very important to me, and if you tell me good things about myself, I'll be a better lover. To all the men out there, don't be idiots. If you tell a woman she's fat, she won't want to have sex with you."

DECADES OF DESIRE:
THE TWENTIES

Interviewing women in their twenties about sexual desire gives you an appreciation for the word *experimentation*. More than that, it highlights just how much of a transformative decade this is for female sexual development.

The diverse sexual histories of our spokeswomen in this decade make easy generalizations impossible, but a few commonalities emerge. As a group, they are fresh, beautiful, assured and occasionally wise beyond their years. They can talk easily of hookups, "sampling" lovers, threesomes and porn, but each interviewee—in one form or another—quickly expresses contentment at having passed the uninhibited, experimental phase of her evolving sexuality. It seems that a significant attitude adjustment about sex is par for the course in this decade.

"I hear girls in their younger twenties in the bathrooms at clubs talking about wanting to hook up with some guy," says Kathleen, now 28 and enjoying a four-year relationship. "And I'm thinking I am *so glad* I'm not there, so glad I'm not still in that dating, sampling pool. I did that, and at the time it was fun, sure. But now, getting older, I'm wanting to focus on more important things. I think that when I'm in a consistent, one-person, committed relationship, I am able to focus and grow and build on discovering my own self and my own true sexuality."

Today, Kathleen is adamantly opposed to reentering that dreaded dating pool: "I always say if my boyfriend and I break up, I'll be single for the rest of my life, and perfectly happy with my vibrator."

"Whereas men want one-night stands, that's harder for women," suggests Jenna, a spirited redhead who just turned 30. "My desire comes from getting to know someone and wanting to eventually explore that sexually. I want there to be a connection. I'm checking them out as a possible relationship."

Carrie, an attractive, 26-year-old massage therapist and bartender, did most of her experimentation between the ages of 20 and 23, but is happy now to be in a relationship of almost two years.

"I didn't like sleeping around. I'm a relationship girl," she says. "I'm not like Samantha Jones on *Sex and the City*. I like commitment. I like the passionate feeling one guy can give me over and over again. Now I just want one person."

Michelle, a 23-year-old lesbian engaged to her partner of 4½ years, expresses a similar gratitude for a stable relationship.

"I'd take a long-term relationship over a one-night stand anytime, absolutely," she says. "Knowing I have a future with the person I'm with now is what stimulates my desire. We're getting married; we're going to have children, buy a house. It's not like high school, when you're with other people. That's nothing like what real passion and love can do in the bedroom."

GETTING STARTED

The one married woman in our group of interviewees—Keisha, a 29-year-old elementary school teacher—reports the least amount of "sampling." Her early sexual encounters involved oral sex only, twice when she was the performer and three times when she was on the receiving end but did not reciprocate. She had an unpleasant introduction to intercourse—at 18—and didn't try it again until a year later, when she became sexually active with the man who's now been her husband for five years.

"It hurt," she recalls of that single, initial encounter. "My overall impression was, 'That was just awful.' No one said I was going to bleed. I thought he broke something. I guess I had sex with him for curiosity's sake. You know, everyone's doing it and it seems like the thing. It sounds so wonderful. Then . . . blood everywhere! They don't talk about that. I didn't know what I was doing. I really didn't."

After that, Keisha retreated from sexual activity until she began dating her future husband after graduation.

Michelle also describes a less-than-ideal initiation to sex [the man already had a girlfriend and hid it from her to get her into bed], but others in their twenties report no trauma with their first encounter, and indicate that curiosity was often a factor in their decision to have intercourse. In general, our interviewees in this age group did not prove to be particularly early arrivals to the game, sexually speaking. While Michelle lost her virginity (to a man ten years her senior) at age 15, two others had intercourse for the first time at age 18, one was 17 and another was 16½.

Carrie, who was 16½ her first time, thought it was a big deal to wait that long, since she'd been dating the guy since she was 14.

"I snuck into his house by the side door; his parents were on other side of the house. I must have been planning it, because I had made a sex CD with sexy, long songs . . . like Dave Matthews.

I wanted to so bad. I wanted to build it up. I told myself I would wait till I was 16, and I'd made my goal. I was ready mentally."

Kathleen was a junior in high school when she and her boyfriend had sex. They had dated for six months, and she chose Valentine's Day for her deflowering.

"I thought, 'Why not.' There was no burning desire. I could have gone six more months. Actually, we tried and it didn't happen. I was tight and it wasn't going to happen. He was sweet and said, 'We can just try tomorrow,' but I got my period and we had to wait a week. I remember it hurting, but it wasn't anything excruciating. It felt really tight. Looking back, it was not good at all. I only hope he's gotten better with time."

THE BIG PICTURE

A look at the 20-something survey takers shows that kissing and touching (with the neck area mentioned frequently) are high on their lists of sexually stimulating behavior, as is their partner's desire for them. Twelve percent—of the 145 respondents in this decade—say "just seeing him" is all it takes, while almost 7 percent mention erotic books, porn or sexy movies in this category. And women this age make numerous references to emotional attachment as a key component to their desire.

What is a 20-something woman thinking about during sex? "How much I love him" is a frequent answer, with a few "Am I doing this right?" and "Is he enjoying this?" responses. About 12 percent are wondering whether they'll have an orgasm or are trying to keep their minds clear so they *can* orgasm. But the largest number—almost 40 percent—say they are in the moment and feeling good. Women in this decade are routinely able to focus on the pleasure at hand, though 6 percent say their to-do lists occasionally pop up, especially when the sex isn't good or they're not into it.

During sex, another 18 percent of 20-somethings are thinking about pleasing their partner or making the experience better in some way, giving credence to their reputation as enthusiastic experimenters. This pleasure-enhancing statistic drops to 9 percent for women in their thirties and 14 percent for those in their forties. A few 20-something women are debating how much information to share with their partner about what they like: They may be thinking, "Touch me here," but aren't able to voice their desire. There's also some genuine wondering: "Why does oral give me orgasm and not his penis?" writes one woman.

Almost 5 percent of 20-somethings (the highest for any decade) are worried about their bodies and how they look during sex, illustrating their evolving self-esteem. One woman wonders whether her lover thinks she's fat; another says, "I hope my partner isn't thinking about someone else."

More than half (56 percent) in this age group say their quickest route to orgasm is either oral sex or some unspecified form of clitoral stimulation. A dozen women (of 145) name vibrators as their top choice, and 13 specify that manual clitoral stimulation works best. Another 13 women cite penetration as their quickest route, and several say it's difficult for them to reach orgasm at all.

As for the biggest lie they were told, almost half the women left this question blank or said they were never lied to. Of those who cited a lie, the largest percentage by far—almost 30 percent—say it was being told that sex is the best thing ever and orgasms are easy to come by. Their comments reinforce that first times aren't always good and in fact sometimes hurt. Several say they believe it takes experience to make things work, and our in-depth interviews bore this out. Other "lies" include debunked myths about how to keep from getting pregnant, and being told you should wait till marriage to engage in sex.

SPECIFICS, PLEASE

The general survey doesn't delve into a woman's total number of partners, her frequency of sex, percentage of orgasms or even her age at first intercourse, but our in-depth interviews uncover all such details. As noted, our 20-something interviewees began sexual relations between ages 15 and 18, which was somewhat later than the teens we interviewed (who started as early as 13), and similar to the women in their thirties, although a few in that decade waited for sex until their mid-twenties.

As for number of partners, the span extends from two (the aforementioned Keisha) to 13 (both Kathleen and bartender Carrie give this total). Michelle had 11 male lovers before settling down with the first female partner she had sex with. Jenna says she's been with five partners.

Frequency of orgasm is above 50 percent for all the 20-something women we spoke with.

Jenna, who enjoyed a 10-year relationship with her first boyfriend, says she's "pretty lucky" and has orgasms 90 percent of the time. She attributes this to being open to trying new things in the bedroom, being honest and having a good mentor for her first lover.

She and her boyfriend were 15 when they met, and they waited almost three years to have sex.

"Everything we did with each other was the first," she recalls, "even our first kiss. We progressed from making out to fingers to oral, but we waited. We were struggling with our upbringing and church teachings. That was all that was keeping us from doing it. And then we decided, 'You know what? We want that first time to be fireworks.' So we went on a nice vacation to Disney and lost our virginity to each other."

The frequency of their coupling varied, depending on what was going on in their lives. "Sometimes we would be like animals and go for it every night, and sometimes there would be a couple weeks until we engaged in sexual activity. When we had our downtimes it actually made us recognize how much we enjoyed our sex life. And soon after that epiphany we would make sure to make time for intimate moments."

Keisha, who usually has sex with her husband four times a week, reports orgasms about half the time. The other half is when she's not in the mood, but has sex anyway for her partner.

"You know, you just do what you gotta do and go to sleep. [To orgasm] I have to focus and get in the mind-set. Sometimes I think they really don't need us; it just takes a magazine and their right or left hand. I'm jealous. It just takes so much more for me."

Keisha has very few orgasms through oral sex; instead, being on top is her surest bet.

"I'm picturing a romantic setting so I can finish; I'm kind of in the zone. Right then I'm not thinking of pleasing my partner. When I'm on top, it's all about me."

Oral sex, she notes, is just a jumping-off point for the couple's usual routine. Then they progress to doggy style—"he has to get that in"—or perhaps missionary.

"Then it's oral on me again and then I'll get on top," she says. "I finish and then I'm just done. I honestly zone out. I could be reading a book. He might take another 15 minutes before he has an orgasm. He lasts a long time, even longer when he's drinking. He can last forever. I can't deal with that."

Keisha is in the majority, according to Dr. Whelihan: Most

women—especially married ones—don't require marathon lovemaking sessions. The general consensus is that ten or fifteen minutes of penetration is plenty, and that it should occur after the woman has had an orgasm.

When Keisha is having her period, the couple's weekly sex schedule falls to zero.

"I get my week off," she says. But normally they have sex all three nights of the weekend and then perhaps Wednesday as well.

"If we go a long time without it, we have to do it three days in a row, which sucks." Keisha laughs. "Because I'm good; I've had an orgasm and can be good for a few days. I'm really not into that mood anymore. I'm satisfied after one day or night. I'm good, but unfortunately, not him. I don't know how they build up so much sexual energy."

Frequency varies among couples, of course, and Dr. Whelihan points out that the parameters for normal libido are wide.

"It's *normal* for an individual to want sex once a month; we call that low drive," she says. "The high-drive individual wants sex daily, and the average individual wants it once a week. It is important that young women recognize their natural drive so that they do not overexpress their interest and mislead their partner. Realize that most individuals can be more sexually active than their normal drive given the correct stimulus: i.e., frequent kissing, passionate chase, flowers, etc. Most of these extra stimuli go away once the relationship continues, which allows the person to revert to their normal pattern."

Based on the anecdotal responses of women in her practice, Dr. Mo says around 20 percent of women fall into the "high" range described above, another 20 percent are "low" and the rest make up the once-or-twice-a week category.

ANOTHER "NORMAL"

Kathleen, a petite blonde with multiple piercings, says she and her lover Don have sex once or twice a week, "though he would like it a lot more."

But she has three jobs and a hectic schedule. Since one of those jobs is as a dancer at a downtown club, it seems reasonable to request a few details on how that might affect her desire.

"I know I am nightly masturbatory material for men," she shares. "If I think about it, it'll completely disgust me. I'm dancing half-naked and these men are obviously fucking me in their mind. If I think about it too much it's really off-putting, that I really am a sex object. I'm part of that glorification of sex; I'm part of that market. But it's easy money. I do think you have to have thick skin and be strong-minded to do it, because they are stripping you in their mind. If I'm walking through the club and a guy grabs my ass, that comes with the job. If it's truly inappropriate, then you get a bouncer, but I work at a good place where there are not a lot of jerks."

Kathleen began having sex at age 17 and experienced her first orgasm three or four years later. Now, when she and Don have sex, oral sex is almost always a part of their routine, and Kathleen says she has orgasms 100 percent of the time when he gives her oral sex.

"He loves to go down on me," she says. "Loves, loves, loves it. Even when we were just friends, I knew him as a guy who was just a freak for vaginas. He's so shocked when he talks to other guys who won't go down, because he's just crazy obsessed. Seriously. He'll beg me some days to go down on me. He's really good at it and he's really eager. I lucked out in that department."

Kathleen is currently off birth control pills because of her history with migraine headaches, so she and Don use condoms, which she says affects her ability to orgasm.

"I can still orgasm during penetration with my boyfriend [when she's on top], but it does take more work and it's less intense when I do."

A late bloomer, Kathleen says she refers to herself as "broken," because her desire for sex was low for so long.

"When I was younger, I wasn't connected to my sexuality at all. I was the ugly duckling. . . . I had no positive attention from guys till the end of high school. That's when I came out of my tomboy/braces/glasses/awkward phase. When I started getting positive attention from guys, it was such a new thing. Even kissing was weird; I wasn't familiar with it. When I started having sex, I just wanted the positive physical attention from guys. It was amazing to me that a guy would want to have sex with me. It wasn't about me; it was about the guy."

When she became intimate with her current boyfriend, at about age 24, Kathleen felt she finally gained control over her sexuality.

"When I first discovered I could have an orgasm on top, it was great! Something all women want to achieve is orgasm with penetration—that is what's 'supposed' to happen. I'd heard it was this unattainable thing, and I thought I couldn't. [But then I learned] it was something I could totally control and I achieved this unachievable orgasm through penetration. When compared to thinking I was 'broken,' it was great to discover I could orgasm from all these other ways, even intercourse. It was empowering, totally."

She's not the only 20-something with such struggles. For Michelle, who finds it challenging to orgasm, deception became the norm.

"I got so good at faking it that it was ridiculous," says the

23-year-old lesbian who dated men for several years before meeting her partner. "All I did was fake it. I didn't have an orgasm unless I gave it to myself."

For satisfaction, she used her fingers; until she met her partner more than four years ago, she didn't own a vibrator.

"It's actually pretty hard to get me off," she shares. "I don't know if I'm extra difficult or what the problem is. It takes both interior stimulation and clit for the most part. Of course, there are always those heated moments that it doesn't matter."

In fact, the first time Michelle engaged in heavy petting with her current lover, she achieved several orgasms.

"We were both fully clothed, in bed, just on each other, grinding, and I got off three or four times that night because it was so intense with a woman. Maybe it was because I had been so deprived from not getting off with men, but I was thrilled I could get off with my clothes on."

These days, Michelle's quickest route to orgasm is a Rabbit vibrator, which provides the dual stimulation she desires and enables her to achieve multiple orgasms.

Her sexual experience with men leads her to speculate on gender differences: "For some reason guys never wanted to go that extra step to try to please me," she says. "Women go that extra step. You can tell with each other, you know, if you've hit a good spot, if you're getting close. . . . I don't know if it's because women just know or because [my partner and I] have been together so long. But women actually care."

Carrie experienced her first orgasm courtesy of a vibrator, and remembers she was about 18 at the time—and alone. She didn't have orgasms with partners until she was 22, with a 19-year-old virgin she says was her twelfth lover.

"It was a summer fling," she says. "Very thrilling and exciting."

She didn't orgasm from penetration, though she was on top. "It lasted about two minutes, which is pretty good for a virgin." She laughs. "We fooled around after and he wanted me to get off. I said, 'All right, this is how it's done.' I showed him. I feel the guy needs to be able to do it himself; plus they like the idea of watching you do it. He got me off with his fingers. But you know, he never went down on me. He wanted me to go down on him, and I would, because I like it. I never asked him to [reciprocate]. He was into his own experience of sex, you know? Not 'together sex.'"

With her current partner, Carrie says she has orgasms about 80 percent of the time. Of those, maybe half occur as she masturbates during penetration and the other half are from penetration alone or her lover masturbating her before or after intercourse.

"I'm over trying to find my G-spot, trying to find what gets me off, because I know I can take care of it later. I love taking care of my man first. And he *does* take care of me, but it's not a priority [for me] to get off every time. If I'm hot and heavy, then I can let go and breathe and get into it. But if [the desire] is not there at the start, it's very hard for me to get into it. If I'm hungry, I might be thinking about what I'm going to eat. 'Do I have that in my fridge?'"

When Carries uses her fingers to achieve orgasm, she says it's generally a quick process, taking a couple of minutes.

"And within thirty seconds, I can have another," she says. "Sometimes it's a fun game. He likes watching. We'll see how many I can do, until I say, 'Okay, I'm tired.' I've been to eleven, back-to-back."

TESTING THE EQUIPMENT

Experimentation is a key to the behavior of women in their

early twenties, with many settling down to a single partner by decade's end. For this age group, what exactly do those years of research look like and lead to? Jenna offers an articulate account of her journey.

"At this point, everything is figured out; I'm an open book," she says. "Right from the get-go I'll tell you what I want and don't want. I'm not afraid to express my sexual needs, my sexual wants. My parents raised me to try food at the dinner table; I didn't have to like it, but I did have to try it. I brought that philosophy to the bedroom and I've tried a lot, and I've found out there's little that I don't like."

From the beginning, Jenna kept an open mind. When her boyfriend of several years wanted to give her oral sex, she initially struggled with the idea.

"He said, 'I'd like to go down on you,' and I was like, 'Oh, I don't know, I don't know. Are you sure you wanna do that?' He said, 'Absolutely.' And the first time he did it, I could feel myself about to have an orgasm, but I didn't think I should. [Oral sex] didn't feel sexually interesting to me, but it was to him, so I did it for his sake and I found out I loved it."

Because the couple was together for more than a decade, Jenna found it important to mix things up to avoid losing passion or becoming bored.

"His libido was stronger than mine, so because I'm open and want to try things, he was like my mentor in the bedroom. And because I'd been with him for so long, I wasn't afraid. I was always interested in what we could do to make the best sexual connection. And he wasn't afraid I'd find something disgusting. We'd talk about it before."

For instance, he introduced porn, but not in an insistent way.

"He might say, 'Do you want to watch this? We don't have to.'

I'd like if it was on in the background, not the focus, where we'd be having some wine and giggling or flirting. Then maybe we'd catch something out of the corner of our eye and he'd ask, 'Is that something you would like?'"

Jenna found porn to be a comfortable way to gather ideas or be introduced to a new concept. Then she would add her own touch.

"I wanted to do my part to keep myself up and keep him interested. He was a good-looking guy and as we went into college, a lot of girls were interested in him. I wanted to make sure I did my part so he wanted to go home with me. I knew when we went home, I could bring it in the bedroom, and we could have that connection there. I wanted to continue to grow with him sexually."

Jenna maintains there is no "one time" in her life when sex was the best; instead her best encounters occur sporadically when she takes a negative situation or transforms an innocent moment into a hot sexual situation that makes for memorable lovemaking. For instance, in a private cubicle at an amusement park, she brought to life a scenario she fantasizes about to this day.

"As quick as I said, 'Wouldn't it be fun to do a quickie?' in a photo booth, his pants were around his ankles and I was on his lap. It's not necessarily when you're in some contorted position, but taking an unexpected moment and making it a hot, sexy moment. That's the best."

In the bedroom, Jenna says she enjoys watching the action in mirrors, especially lately, with a new partner.

"I like it from behind with a smack on the ass, but I also like it on top, when I'm pressed hard against him, with one of his hands on my ass cheek. In the [13 years] I've been sexually active, there have been times where it's penetration [I enjoy most] and times where it's oral sex. That's why I like mixing it up; I never know when that phase is going to change. Currently it's watching, from behind and on top, with him pulling me close. But there have definitely been times in my life when I come into a phase where oral sex is what I'm craving. I luckily have multiple orgasms, but sometimes I want the first orgasm to be from oral sex and the next one to be from penetration."

Her adventuresome attitude is something Jenna plans never to lose: "I've evolved from a person coming of age in the college sex scene, where it's a free-for-all, with threesomes and girls kissing girls and all of that, to now, when I think of getting married and having kids. So now my interest and body will change, but I'm willing to change with it. I'm willing to explore and dive into whatever's next. I hear from married people how awful the sex becomes, and I don't understand why that has to happen. I understand that things change, but I have the ability to have multiple orgasms and I don't want a kid or anything to change that. I want to continue to explore and have desires."

A BIT OF DRESS-UP

Like Jenna, Keisha is a fan of porn, and though she once watched with her girlfriends, now she enjoys solo viewing. She prefers heterosexual videos and doesn't masturbate while watching, preferring to "play later" with her husband, Tony.

To keep things interesting sexually, they shop at adult lingerie stores and role-play often.

"We started right after we got married; we used to do it every other weekend. His role-playing choice is always in a strip club and I'm the stripper and doing the dancing and then we go have sex. We got a strobe light, the stripper shoes, music—the whole deal. Mostly we do his [fantasy]. Mine is a little cornier:

We pretend we don't know each other, get to know each other, see where it goes. I like to build more of a history behind my story. He tries to be someone else, but he does an awful job." She laughs.

Their experience gives credence to the conventional wisdom that men are more commonly aroused by simple visual stimulation, while women may prefer a sexy romance novel or more detail-laden fantasies.

Tony is very handsome and Keisha says his body "is ridiculous; he keeps it so nice." This increases her sexual desire for him, though the difference in their visual cues is again apparent.

"It annoys me that he looks at the mirror when we're having sex," she reveals. "It makes me feel dirty. I'm not sure why. It doesn't feel right . . . like he's making a show out of it."

Other areas of the couple's sex life are very satisfying for Keisha; for instance, they have little games they play to prolong the anticipation of sex.

"I realize, with me, it turns me on when I don't give in to him easily. Like, he'll go to grab my boob, and I say, 'No, no, you can't touch me.' Then he says, 'You know you like it,' and I'll deny it. It's fun. It goes all the way until we're having sex. We've been doing that for a while; we play it till we're actually having sex. It's the chase. I do enjoy that."

When does the game end?

"When the panties come off, the door's open." She laughs. "If the panties are still on, he has to work for it. That's the motto."

THE FURTHER ADVENTURES OF THE TWENTIES

Carrie, the massage therapist and bartender, is happy in her current two-year relationship with a man 14 years her senior. But she admits the best sex of her life was on a water tower one night during her summer fling when she was 22.

She had five orgasms that night and says "crazy sex" was a hallmark of the summer. "We had it everywhere—on a washing machine while it was going . . . it was fantasy sex every time. But I was a lot more emotionally involved than he was."

When they broke up, Carrie says her desire fell and her sex drive went into neutral.

"My hormones weren't raging. I would kiss guys, but was I dry; I didn't have anything going on. So I talked to Dr. Whelihan and I remember she said, 'You haven't found the right guy you want to have sex with.' She said, 'Don't worry; it'll come. You'll get horny. You'll get wet.'

"And she was right. With [my summer fling] it was good sexually, but we weren't aligned otherwise. With the guy now, it's *all* good. I'm wet all the time and uncontrollable. I experimented dating multiple guys, long-term, short-term; I think I've covered the scale pretty well. But now I just want one person. That's my desire. That's what I've desired for 10 years."

Not that Carrie doesn't still experiment. In fact, she says she's learned more from her boyfriend than from anyone else.

"Because we trust each other, we're open to trying new things. I'm unafraid to tell him what I want, and he tells me what he wants, and if it's totally crazy we'll laugh, but we'll try it. There are no inhibitions. I've never had that before. Talking about things with my partner, I just learn so much every day. Like he asks me, 'What makes you feel sexy?' Last night we played strip blackjack. We love blackjack, and we're always trying to think of something new. So we'd take something off or do something sexy for the winner. It was fun. And with a glass of wine you never know what'll happen!

"When I was dating around, I think I *thought* I learned a lot, because of the 'practice.' But I was only learning things on the surface. [Now I have a] partner I want to do everything with, sexual and nonsexual. I love him. I think I've learned the most in this deep relationship."

Michelle, at 23 the youngest of this decade's spokeswomen, experimented with her sexuality in a big way, finding she was oriented to women after a series of dissatisfying relationships with men. It surprised even her.

"My sister is gay," she explains. "When I was underage, she got me a fake ID and would let me drink with her so she could keep tabs on me. The only place we ever went was gay clubs. That was fine with me; I was friends with all her friends. I always said, 'There's nothing wrong with being gay; it's just not for me.' And that was pretty much my attitude till I met my partner. I thought other girls could do stuff to me, but I wouldn't be able to please them. I had kissed other girls before and had developed crushes, but nothing that was long-lasting or sexual. I wasn't really looking for something, but I had opened up to the possibility because I'd never been pleased by a man and I thought that was maybe why."

Though her partner has had threesomes with men and women, Michelle says she has no desire for that.

"My partner knows I wouldn't be game whatsoever."

But she does enjoy experimenting and tells a story of using her Rabbit vibrator in the car late one night, when she was in the passenger seat and her partner was driving. Asking her partner to warn her if someone passed in another vehicle, Michelle tipped the seat back and lost herself in the moment.

"I kept going and had four, five or six orgasms! When I opened my eyes, we were stopped at red light in a small town! It was 3 in morning but I was still freaked out and pulled my skirt down and said, 'Why didn't you make me stop?' She said, 'Well, you were enjoying yourself and I was enjoying watching.'"

The threesomes Michelle dismisses appeal to one of our 20-somethings: Kathleen and her partner, Don, have recently participated in two such encounters, both times with women from their group of friends.

"I never thought I'd ever have an attraction to women," Kathleen says, "and I still don't think I do. Growing up, there were girls experimenting, bisexual, [but] I was totally uninterested; I couldn't imagine going down on another girl. The first time we did it, it was insane. It was a really organic process. We had been drinking a lot and I think alcohol played a big part, because your insecurities and inhibitions go down. It becomes not such a taboo thing.

"Anyway, it was the three of us and she was dancing around. She pulled her top down and Don said, 'You have Kathleen's nipples! Kathleen, take your top down!' It turned into touching and kissing and petting. . . . It was very organic, very cool. You think it's gonna be awkward, like, 'What do I do when this person is doing this?' but with the three of us, it was just this flowy, organic kissing. Later on, Don and I set up rules, and decided if this was to ever happen again, he wouldn't want a guy in the threesome, and I wouldn't want him to have intercourse with another girl. I'm fine with him going down on her, but I don't know how I'd feel if the other girl went down on him. He said me going down on the other girl was the hottest thing he'd ever seen. She went down on me too. He loved watching these other girls as into me as he is into me."

Since both parties enjoyed the experience, a follow-up to the threesome was arranged.

"The second time was with another girlfriend who Don

always said had a girl crush on me. It happened after some drinks. I remember walking into my house and them both ripping my clothes off. That time was even better, because she was a lot older and she was so sexual. She was in her early thirties. The other woman had been in her early twenties. This one had more of a grip on her sexuality. She was experienced and a lot more sensual. She knew we'd had a threesome before. I told her she blew [the other girl] out of the water. I thought the first was great, but the second time was even better. I was just discussing with Don how nice it is that three people can come together like this. We're all responsible adults; it's this innocent thing. We can experience our own and each other's sexuality and enjoy it. And not feel that it's some crazy, dirty, taboo act."

AND YET . . .

Experimentation has its limits, it would seem. Of anal sex, Kathleen has this to say: "I hate it. Of the handful of times I've done it, it might have felt okay once. The discomfort is not worth all the effort; it just doesn't feel good. Don jokes and says you won't even feel it. Oh, I feel it! I've tried really hard, but one time it brought me on the verge of tears. I want to make him happy and fulfill his needs too, but there's that fine line where if you're truly uncomfortable, you shouldn't put yourself at risk. I wish that I was one of those who loved it, and I've heard there are women who achieve orgasm through anal sex, but there's just no way."

Other aspects of anal play are okay with Kathleen.

"Don will lick my butt and that's fine; he'll do a finger and that's fine. He's really gentle and he does get it. But it's the girth I can't handle [though she says Don's penis is average]. Is it my favorite? No. It might occasionally feel good, but I could totally live without it."

Neither Keisha nor Michelle has tried anal sex and both say they have no interest. Carrie says she's not a fan but will give it a shot "once in a blue moon," if she's dated the man for a good while.

"I don't mind a finger; fingers are okay. I can handle that. If it's a penis, I don't fare well with it; I just prefer not to."

But most guys Carrie dates either ask every time or try for anal sex, forcing her to get creative. "I will do a little show for him, play around that area. But I just don't get it; I don't get their attraction for it."

Carrie thinks men once equated anal sex with being gay, but now believes straight guys have viewed porn depicting heterosexual anal sex so often that "they think it's fine."

Decade-wide, 14.5 percent of 20-something women named anal sex as their top grievance; Jenna, our 30-year-old redhead, is the only in-depth interviewee in this decade to advocate for the practice.

"I'm not crazy about [anal sex], but with clitoral stimulation I've found I can come to orgasm that way, so I'm willing to try it. I can see that I might come to a place where vaginal penetration doesn't do it for me and maybe [anal] would."

She even offered tips for first-timers who are curious about the experience.

"Start with oral on your ass, or fingers or small toys," she says. "Get comfortable with that area of your body and the idea of it not just being exit-only. Work yourself up to it; it's not something that you just take nine inches from behind.

"It's not such an attraction for us, but it is for guys, who are visual. And yes, it is a tight area that is uncomfortable from the start. For me, it requires a lot of alcohol. It kills the inhibition and allows you to relax. But initial entry *is* tight. The person you're with can't just plow you. He should want it to be as enjoy-able for you as for himself. If he sees it's getting uncomfortable, he should back up, maybe go back to fingers or vibrators. Let [the process] evolve to you wanting him to put it there."

Even with preparation, anal sex can be uncomfortable for women.

"I did all those things and the initial entry was still a bit of a shock," Jenna says. "I found that clitoral stimulation [with fingers or a vibrator] takes away some of the painful attention to that initial entry and turns it into a pleasurable distraction."

In summary, Jenna advises women that their answer to a request for anal sex doesn't have to be, "Absolutely not."

"You might not like anal sex, but you might like having your ass licked. Open your mind to exploring the anal area. You don't know what you might discover."

TRANSFORMATIONAL TWENTIES

At first, the twenties decade seemed a bit schizophrenic, but it was only because the women made such large shifts in their attitudes and opinions about sexuality during that time span. Their stories prove that while the early twenties seem to be a time for in-the-moment living and enjoying the freedom to experiment, just a few years later these same women tend to adopt the cultural norms of a monogamous relationship and all that comes with it.

While they don't actually repudiate their pasts, by age 27 or 28 our interviewees had mostly discarded the sexual lifestyle of their early twenties, shifting from a day-to-day existence to projecting toward a future with one partner.

As Kathleen says: "Sampling was fun, but did it mean any-thing? No. It was just for the time."

These women loved their periods of experimentation, but by decade's end they are already learning some of the basic tenets of what women will tell us more about as they get older: i.e., they like other lovers, but it's generally best with one guy or girl. After an enthusiastic embrace of experimentation, many 20-something women discover that monogamy and more traditional sexual practices suit them.

Nevertheless, they all seem to understand that an ability to spice it up in the bedroom is crucial to maintaining a satisfying sexual relationship.

DECADES OF DESIRE:
THE THIRTIES

AH, YES, THE INFAMOUS THIRTIES. THE TIME IN A WOMAN'S LIFE when legend has it she is enjoying her sexual peak. She's past the awkwardness of her youth, experiencing the blush of physical beauty and relishing her ability to chart her own course in the bedroom.

Dr. Whelihan confirms that women in their thirties have "emerging confidence, good physical fitness, stable hormones, overall good health and a youthful marriage/relationship, all of which packages nicely into a decade of great sexual satisfaction."

And among our 165 survey respondents in this decade, we did indeed find many sexually satisfied women. Our in-depth interviews uncovered Anna, a 39-year-old wife who never fails to achieve orgasms during lovemaking sessions with her husband of 12 years; Cyndi, a cheerful bisexual of 32 who rarely turns down sex and—since she turned 25 and "figured things out"—enjoys orgasms 90 percent of the time; and Emily, a 35-year-old single woman who became sexually active at 20 and now has orgasms with every encounter. "I've had 16 partners exactly," she shares. "It wasn't until I was 30 that the number skyrocketed; that's when it doubled. It's amazing what they say about the thirties. I feel like a guy; I'm ready to go anytime."

Dr. Whelihan attributes this decade's healthy sex drive to a happy confluence of circumstances.

"Although many are married with children, the marriage is still fresh and exciting and the kids are manageable, so there's a little less stress than in other decades," she says. "In addition, women this age are less likely to be managers and CEOs, so there's not that professional pressure to perform at the peak of their ability. Plus, their bodies are still young; very few have major medical problems, and they are still enjoying the ease of maintaining a youthful body. Finally, the thirties ladies enjoy adequate, stable hormone levels and therefore are less affected by the mood swings and menstrual drama often seen as we transition into the forties."

In fact, 26 percent of our surveyed women in their thirties indicate they *are* having the best sex of their lives "right now." (This compares with 16.5 percent of 40-something women and 13 percent of 50-somethings who say they are currently having the best sex of their lives.)

But that assessment by a quarter of the 30-somethings must be balanced against the 17 percent of women in this decade who say they are still waiting for their best sex. (In addition, 13 percent of women in this decade say the biggest lie they were told about sex is that it's always great.)

So perhaps some of the general satisfaction of the thirties is attributable to simply attaining a perspective in life where one is inclined to look back and assess—while still having the attractiveness, physical mobility and curiosity for experimentation to make the most of every sexual encounter.

Our in-depth interviews encompassed married, single and divorced women, including one bisexual and a closeted lesbian.

While their levels of lust are vastly dissimilar, one thing they share is clarity about who they are and how they've arrived at their current location in the desire continuum. Thirty-something women still have issues to sort out, but they tend to understand the emotional undercurrents that affect their sex drive and see clearly the paths they've traveled.

Mickey, for instance, knew exactly how she wanted her sex life to change when she found a new boyfriend after ending her 16-year marriage to a man she describes as controlling and jealous, albeit a good lover.

"I was always afraid to wound their ego by telling [a guy] what I liked," says the petite redhead. "After my divorce, I wanted to make my new relationship with my boyfriend better, but they take it personally when you speak up, like you don't like *them*. How's it going to be good for both of you if he doesn't get that there has to be communication? My husband destroyed my sex drive; he told me I lay there like a bump on a log. He'd say, 'Why don't you want me like I want you?' I wanted to say, 'Because you want sex and I want a relationship.' I mean, we had a relationship, sure, but he never made me feel special, like I was in his thoughts that day or that he really cared what was happening to me."

Mickey, 37, lost her virginity at 15, and became pregnant by her future husband—her third lover—while a senior in high school.

"I used to dread sex with my husband because it was for satisfying his desires," she recalls. "He was good at satisfying mine too, but I didn't crave it; I didn't want it. I never wanted sex, really. I guess it stems from the guilty feelings that came when I started [having sex] as a teenager and really didn't want to."

Like many women interviewed for this book, Mickey had

sex her first time not as a capitulation to overwhelming lust or desire, but because it felt like the assumed—and certainly expected—progression in the dating game.

She had been dating her high school boyfriend for 10 months and agreed to sex "because I thought that was the next step in the relationship. I thought he was going to break up with me if I didn't. I had a lot of guilt; I'd gone to church all my life and thought, 'I shouldn't be doing this; my Mom and Dad are going to be mad at me.' I felt I was going to let them down and not meet their expectations as a Christian."

Mickey remembers the experience as a letdown; one she "didn't get much feeling from." Adding a sexual component didn't radically change her relationship with her boyfriend, and she continued to feel guilty.

"He knew I was a virgin and that I wasn't really ready," she says. "But we both loved each other, so I didn't have a fear that I'd be used or hurt or that he'd leave me afterward."

Mickey ended that relationship at 16, and started another soon after with a handsome football star who began pressuring her for sex right away. She gave in, but knew "he was just going through the girls" as fast as possible. They parted when she discovered he was smoking pot and seeing a girl in another town, but she says it took her many years to get over the infatuation.

At the end of her junior year, Mickey met her future husband, Frank, an older guy who was 23. He took her to the junior prom, and once again she felt pressured to put out.

"In a small town, everyone has boyfriends," she explains. "That's all there is to do: no bowling alley, no movie theater, no skating rink."

Though she gave in on prom night, Mickey was racked with guilt.

"I told him, 'I've already been with two guys; we can't start doing this.' I wanted to wait to get married [this time]. He said, 'You can't do that. You can't give it to me and then stop.' So I felt pressured again, for the third time."

But Frank was different in two important ways: He didn't use condoms and he wanted Mickey to have orgasms.

"The first two guys always wore condoms," she says. "With Frank, he thought he knew better. He said he would pull out—and he did, but the pre-cum got me pregnant."

Frank also made sure Mickey experienced her first orgasm, during oral sex.

"He was a lot older and knew I wasn't having orgasms, and he was like, 'We're going to do this until you have it.' He was determined; he thought I was missing out on something. But I knew what he offered, and I didn't care to be having it. It's not that I didn't want to have orgasms; it's that I didn't want to have sex, because I didn't feel close to him. He didn't make me feel special."

And while she's quite happy with her current boyfriend, two decades later Mickey occasionally wonders if she retains a few vestiges of her early sexual behavior.

"Sometimes I read articles or something where women talk about sex, and I think maybe I'm not getting out of it what they're getting. When I'm really into it, it feels good, but it's never that thing people say, like, '*Oh, my god!* This feels *so* good. I can't *wait* for that again!' For me, it's like, 'Oh, that's nice,' or, 'This is a good position.'"

LIFE AFTER ABUSE

Tonya, a 39-year-old married mother of two, has had a rockier terrain of sexual history to navigate, but like Mickey, she can clearly articulate the path she's traveled. She credits years of therapy—beginning in college—for helping her deal with long-term childhood sexual abuse and confront her homosexuality.

"I think the abuse defined my sexuality, unfortunately," she admits. "I was introduced to sex much too early in life: too early, too often, by too many people."

At age 13, Tonya put a stop to the abuse she'd endured by hysterically insisting she would tell the family if her abuser ever touched her again. But nothing could stop the repercussions.

"I do think my thinking is . . . I don't want to say warped, but deviated as far as sexual desires," she shares. "I assume everyone is an abuser instead of giving people the benefit of the doubt. It makes me very untrusting of men.

"I honestly believe some people are born gay and some people have life experiences that can steer them in a different direction," she says. "I think I'm the latter."

Though she kept secret the abuse she feels defines her sexual preferences, Tonya, the youngest of eight children, did find the conviction to come out as gay to her mother and sister during her college years. She believes her mother was shocked at the news, though multiple strokes had robbed the older woman of the ability to speak. Nevertheless, Tonya wanted to be truthful.

"Nobody in my family speaks the word *gay* or *homosexual* unless they're laughing or are picking at someone who's gay," she says. "I had to find my way sexually on my own; there were no talks. Every sexual experience was on my own. The first woman I went out with, I was 18; she was one of my college teachers. That was the first acknowledgment of my homosexuality and the first moment I had the courage to pursue it. Of course I couldn't tell anyone. My life has been one big secret after another."

An educational professional today, Tonya was the sole caretaker of her mother during the final 13 years of her life. Though her mom died when Tonya was 32, she hadn't heard her voice since she was 17 because of the stroke damage.

And in all those years of living together, Tonya never revealed the sexual abuse.

"I never wanted to hurt her. I didn't want her to think she was a bad mom. She was a great mom. She worked really hard. She was never around because she worked so much. I knew telling her would destroy her."

Tonya's abuse began when she was 4, with a onetime molestation by an uncle. Then her stepfather raped her when she was 8.

"I can never forget it. Then my aunt's boyfriend when I was about 10; then some guy in the park one day when I was 11; then my sister's boyfriend for three years when I was in sixth, seventh and eighth grade. It kept recurring over and over again," she recounts wearily.

In fact, Tonya did speak up about her abuse the first time it happened, on a family trip to the country to visit relatives.

"I told because I was 4. When you're 4 you tell everything. It was my uncle and he was a teenager. I told my mom and later she woke me up when Dad got home to tell him what happened. Dad took [my uncle] to the barn and beat him with a tobacco stick."

That was that—and the abuse by that family member stopped. But Tonya's parents continued to send her back to the same relatives every summer, where the abuse eventually resumed with another family member.

"I wouldn't do that to my kids," says Tonya, who refuses to allow her kids to stay overnight anywhere. "But maybe [my folks] thought if I told before, I'd tell again."

Today, Tonya holds her father responsible for much of her past.

"My parents got divorced when I was 7; pretty much everything that happened to me I blame on my dad. Walking away is one thing, but walking away without ever turning around is different. If the men who abused me knew there was someone, another man in my life who would stand up for me and protect me, who'd come back and beat the living crap out of them, it wouldn't have happened. And I told my dad that—for my own well-being."

Despite her limited identification of herself as a lesbian, Tonya was unable to reconcile her homosexual lifestyle with the church doctrine she absorbed growing up. She had consensual sex with a man for the first time at age 28, and married him.

"One of the reasons I got married is because I thought my husband could cure me, save me, change me . . . that I wouldn't be gay anymore."

That hope was soon dashed by her continuing attraction to women, but Tonya is nevertheless determined to stay put.

"If it wasn't for my religious beliefs [Christian], I wouldn't be in a heterosexual marriage," she says. "I don't live from the inside out, because inside my strong desire is to be with women. And now I can't ruin my children's lives and my 11-year marriage. My children's happiness and their development are more important than my desires. I would never be so selfish as to shake up their lives like that. I wouldn't do that to them."

Tonya's husband knows of her leanings; she told him years ago and says that, in all fairness, she should have told him before they married. He did know about the abuse, and accepted it, but today he won't talk about her desire for women.

Several years into her marriage—complicating matters—

Tonya met Betty and the two had a yearlong affair.

"We were hot and heavy for a year," she recalls. "I consider myself hypersexual when it comes to a female; I have high desire for intimacy with a female. When Betty and I were together, literally she'd touch my arm; I'd be like, 'Okay let's go!' Touch my leg, 'Go!' She called me Dude, because I was like a guy. Guys think all touches are for sex, not just for affection."

The two women were together often, but neither husband was the slightest bit suspicious.

"Three, four, five times a week—every chance we got, we'd have sex. It was a sex fest," Tonya says. "But we could just literally kiss all night and be so filled with each other and so happy. We'd go out to dinner and hold hands under the table; that was just the best thing to us."

Tonya acknowledges that the secrecy aspect of the affair may have contributed to its appeal. But her guilty feelings led her to tell her husband of her desire for women, and six months later she found the nerve to confess the affair. He stipulated that she break it off if they were to continue the marriage, which she did.

"I knew it was too good to be true, knew it wasn't going to last," she says. "It was amazing. I've never felt that way before or since, in my heart or physically. That's what keeps drawing me back to her."

Betty told her own husband about the affair as well, and the two women didn't see or speak to each other for seven years.

But Tonya says they recently reconnected through a mutual friend.

"We're just friends; we're not being physical. We resolved in our hearts and minds and word that we wouldn't betray our husbands again. But our feeling is that, if eight years later, we're still desirous of one another and our hearts are still pining, then we feel if we had a chance, we'd have a great relationship. I told her I want to be just two old ladies traveling the world together. I want to scoop her up, take her and do whatever it is we do together."

For now, Tonya is keeping Betty a secret again, worrying that her husband will feel threatened by her communication with her former lover. And she acknowledges that her marriage is better now, because in the past year her husband seems to be trying to be a better companion and partner.

"He was jobless for three years, but still nothing around the house was getting done. I don't know why it took him so long to start listening . . . but he's finally sensing that I have needs [other than sexual] as a wife that he has not been fulfilling. Plus, now he's self-employed."

And, as Tonya discovers, "When everything else gets better, the sex gets better."

As to the particulars of her sex life with her husband, Tonya says that if the couple didn't engage in oral sex, she would never have orgasms.

"He has diabetes; he was diagnosed 10 years ago, and it affects our relationship a lot. We had a rough patch for about two or three years, with very little sex during that time."

Erectile issues due to diabetes keep the couple from having conventional sex, and they have oral sex instead. Penetration, she estimates, is usually about once every two to three months.

"There's never any ejaculation," she clarifies, "just penetration for as long as he can."

Tonya's husband lost his desire for sex when penetration became an issue. Dr. Whelihan offers that both aging and illness can rob men of this primal urge.

"Penetration for men is the masculine expression of their

sexuality," says the doctor. "They believe their role is to provide a firm penis to their partner, and when this no longer occurs, they feel worthless and inadequate."

Sadly, men who experience erectile dysfunction often withdraw from intimacy, and since the frequency of encounters declines, the problem is exacerbated.

Tonya believes lack of sexual interest from her husband partially explains why her affair with Betty occurred.

"I'm not saying it's his fault. When he couldn't penetrate and didn't have desire, I'd try to tell him, 'We're a *couple*.' But he didn't have desire. That's part of why the affair happened. I found someone who's willing to satisfy all my needs. And we genuinely love each other."

SUPERSATISFIED, THANKYOUVERYMUCH

Although she was a late bloomer, having sex for the first time at 26, Anna finds herself happily married to her first lover, Larry. And who knows? Perhaps that late start contributes to her contentment.

Now 54, Larry is 15 years Anna's senior. He was a coworker who was coming off a long-term relationship when the couple began going out. Anna, a cute, dimpled brunette, had no real boyfriends before Larry, only guys she'd had a few dates with. But after just two weeks, she took Larry to her bed.

"I was dating another guy at the same time," she says. "I broke up with the other guy within a week of dating Larry. I trusted him from the beginning; I was so comfortable with him. It was just really nice."

Most of Anna's girlfriends were sexually active by their early twenties, and they would tease her "in a nice way" about not having sex.

"I just wasn't ready," she says without apology. "There's a big trust factor. I still can't believe I'm sleeping in the same bed with another person. That's a huge trust issue right there. You have to feel safe, that he's not going to hurt you while you're sleeping."

Anna, who also confesses to a fear of the dark, adds that perhaps she has a too-vivid imagination. But in the face of all her misgivings, Larry persevered.

"Comfortable is not a bad thing," she says. "On TV, you see them suggest a dangerous guy, or a bad boy. But comfort and trust are what I want. Someone I feel safe with."

Ask how her desire has changed in the 14 years they've been together, and Anna has much to say.

"We do it just as frequently as we ever did," she begins. "It only stops when we're sick or stressed out. It's not every night, but it sure is close. If we don't during the week, we make up for it during the weekend."

Sessions are usually 30 minutes long, and "sometimes we do it just to take the edge off if we're having a bad day; it can help with stress."

She goes on to say she's more open to variety in their sex life now, and while both always enjoyed oral sex—both giving and receiving—they now have incorporated toys, porn and spanking into their lovemaking.

"I've been getting more comfortable the last few years," Anna says. "I've been asking him to spank me now. Or I'll say, 'I want you to hold me down a little bit more.' I'll tell him if it starts hurting and he'll stop."

Anna says love scenes in movies can stimulate her desire, and she and Larry now watch adult films as well.

"He bought a ton of them off craigslist; we have a jillion to go through."

She jokes about needing to find someone to come into their home and clear the porn out if something happens to both of them.

"I don't want my friends thinking of me in that way— 'Ewww, she watches porn with her husband'—but I don't see anything wrong with it, if it's just us two and if it enhances our lovemaking. People seem to have strong feelings about it, but I see it as an addition to the lovemaking."

Often the couple plays porn in the background. "It gets things started," she says, noting that it doesn't always turn her on. "It's more for him."

As mentioned at the beginning of this chapter, orgasms during sex are a foregone conclusion for Anna. However, she does not achieve orgasm through penetration.

"He's superconsiderate," she says of Larry, who makes sure she climaxes through oral sex. "And we also use toys [to help]. It's always me first. I feel so selfish. But he says, 'No, it's okay. You're great.'"

A vibrator is Anna's quickest route to orgasm: "High is a better frequency for me; there's not enough friction or pulsating on low. And the vibrator does have a heat sensor, which is nice sometimes. If he's there and I'm playing with my toy, then it's way better. Not that I'm looking for an audience, but he plays along. Usually he's touching me, so I have both his hands on me *and* the toy—and it's the best sensations. And sometimes he'll play with himself."

Anna says she would never be interested in a threesome, although it's a fantasy of Larry's.

"His favorite is Claudia Schiffer. I say, 'If she'll have you, go for it. Indulge in your fantasy.' It's just a fantasy and it's nothing else. I don't mind if he says another woman is pretty, because I know he loves me."

Just last year, the couple began experimenting with anal sex.

"I always loved being touched there," Anna says, "but he's never pressured me. We're discussing the kinds of toys we could buy [specific to anal sex]. He's talked about it, but he's never guilted me into it. If he did, I'd just hate the idea. He wants to make sure I enjoy it; it only benefits him in the long run."

Anna recalls their forays into this new territory with relish: "I'm very sensitive down there. He says it is incredibly tight and it feels great and he doesn't last long. And he's playing with my clitoris, making sure I'm having the time of my life. I have to be so ready, both mentally and physically. If I'm not, he won't do it."

How does he know she's ready?

That first time, Larry told her, "You were wet everywhere. You were lifting toward me. Your body was asking for it." And Anna remembers thinking, "Wow, that was great," as she had an orgasm while he was inside her and stimulating her clitoris.

But even as her desire for new activities in the bedroom blossoms, Anna doesn't see any one aspect taking over their love life: "Anal sex is something to change things up; it's like a spanking. I don't expect him to spank me all the time. I wouldn't want that."

It's not surprising that Anna's satisfaction sexually pervades other areas of her life.

"Even though I'm older, I'm more comfortable in my skin than I've ever been. I think it's because he accepts me as I am, warts and all. I swear to you, never did I think I'd feel this way about myself. I know he has a lot to do with it. Because he thinks I'm wonderful, it's made me more self-confident. He's made my life so great. He's always there for me. That has a lot to do with how I feel about being with him . . . always."

HAVING IT BOTH WAYS

While Cyndi, at 32, is seven years younger than Anna, she too exhibits the hallmarks of a woman who is both confident in her sexuality, knowledgeable on the subject of her desires and content with the path she's chosen.

On the topic of what stimulates her desire, Cyndi goes against our survey's tide, which tilts heavily toward kissing. (Overall, 23.6 percent of women in this decade mention kissing—the highest of any decade save women in their nineties.)

"For me, it's thinking about having sex in different positions with toys and various people involved. Or having a hand lightly brush over my body. It's not kissing at all," says the athletic, petite blonde. "I'm a visual person, so thinking about people doing it works. I get turned on by watching porn. Sometimes I feel like I'm a dude in that respect. I'm bisexual; I'll go either way. Depending on the year, my sex life can be more one or the other. For the last two years it was all women. Before that, it was all men [when she was engaged and monogamous for seven years].

"When I watch porn, it has to be girl-on-girl for me to get turned on," she continues. "Watching straight sex does not do it for me. I like straight sex; I just don't like to watch it. Women just look more sexual than men in my eyes."

Cyndi says she definitely finds toys such as vibrators stimulating, noting there's something kinky about them that turns her on. She has no desire to be chained or gagged, but admits she enjoys thinking about such things, especially vibrators.

She also likes porn, but usually only when she masturbates.

"I haven't watched with a partner. For me, I guess porn is a replacement for a partner."

Cyndi's adventurous nature didn't find full expression during her twenties.

"The guy I was engaged to wasn't into any different stuff," she says, "so I wasn't able to experience any of that with him. We just had straight sex, which was fine. It was good sex, but nothing crazy. After we broke up, I really started getting experimental. I'm a sexual person and I wanted to try all of this.

"I was always curious about women; my fiancé used to joke that he was marrying a lesbian. At the end, I was trying to incorporate new stuff; I'd ask if he wanted to handcuff me, get edible stuff and eat it off me, toys, anything—I just need sex!"

A year after their breakup, when she was 29, Cyndi had sex with a woman for the first time.

"It blew my mind. I got really turned on. It was at a friend's going-away party, and I met this girl who was hot. I had just broken up with a guy [after a short relationship] who was a douche bag. I was with him for the sex; he was really good-looking. But I was so sick of men right then. And she whispered to me, 'I want to get you alone.' It was like God just gave me a present, put it right in my lap.

"I was nervous. I felt like a teenage boy on my first hookup. Now I know how dudes feel. 'Where do I touch her? Will she like this?' I mean, I know how I like to be touched, but you don't know how another woman likes to be touched."

Cyndi was "out" right from the start, describing the one-night stand as "awesome" to her platonic girlfriend the very next day.

"Sex with men is great," she says, trying to explain the distinction she feels. "It feels good in a physical way, but it doesn't turn me on in my mind as much. I get off because he's going through the motions, but I'm not all hot and heavy. With a woman, I'm already turned on in my mind before the physical happens. Which is *desire*. With guys I don't think I have as much desire. I get turned on because they're touching the right spots, but I don't have the desire in my mind as much."

Cyndi has been with four female partners; two of those encounters fit her criteria for "longer-term," or more than four months.

"It's not nearly as many as I have guys," says Cyndi, who's been with between 30 and 50 lovers. "I'll resort to having sex with a guy because it's easier. Months go by without sex and it's just easier to hook up with a guy than a girl."

Cyndi's first sexual encounter was at 18 with a guy she met at college.

"The first time was lame," she recounts. "I thought, 'This is it? Really? Please tell me this gets better.' I was so disappointed. People make it sound like it's going to be orgasmic every time and it's not at all. Especially when you're young. You don't know what you're doing. That's why they say sex gets better as you get older. You've perfected what turns you on. If you're with a partner, you can direct them. Of course it'll get better; you know more. And some of your inhibitions start sliding away."

Cyndi did not have orgasms with any of her first three partners, whom she met over the period of a year.

"I liked having sex, but I was not blown away," she says. "I was just doing it out of curiosity. But for me, it got better as it went along. By my second and third year, I moved to a new town and went on a spree there. I think I finally got to have an orgasm by guy number four, and I went in search of more of it."

That search has resulted in a total number of lovers Cyndi is conflicted about. "I've had more than 30 lovers; that's when I stopped counting," she says. "I had 30 three years ago and decided, 'I'm not counting anymore; this is depressing.'

"I think a lot of people are pretty judgmental about it. There shouldn't be shame about having that many lovers, but there's such a [reaction] about hooking up with more than *this* number; you hear 'slut' and 'whore'; all of a sudden you're dirty now. That's the mentality people have. I don't want that to transfer over to myself, but sometimes I do. I have to remind myself, 'There's nothing wrong with you. You're clean; you don't have a child; it's okay.' Sometimes I have an inner struggle over that, though."

WHAT'S WITH OUR "NUMBER"?

She's not alone in these concerns. Emily, the single woman with 16 partners, expresses similar misgivings about running up the number of lovers she's accumulated in her lifetime.

"Why do we care about that number?" she asks. "I always did before, but I stopped caring when I got to my thirties. Then I started caring again. It shouldn't matter, but it does . . . I guess for surveys like this. For me, I want to be able to remember every single person; I don't want to go so overboard that I don't have any idea who I've been with or what I've done."

Emily's "friend with benefits" of six years' standing—whom she sees every couple of months or so if she's not dating—helps her deal with potential guilt surrounding her number.

"It's easy because we know what one another likes—and he's a good person. And my number [of lovers] doesn't go through the roof!"

Emily says that number was eight until she entered her thirties, when her libido mushroomed.

"[My desire] has become more intense," she says. "I actually yearn to have sex. Before it was something I did with another person in a relationship."

Today, at 35, she's able to separate sex and relationships.

"I no longer have to have an emotional connection in order to have sex, good sex, any kind of sex," she says, laughing. "To me, all sex is good. It all feels good."

Emily, whose longest relationship was a three-year stint in college, finds men her age are "not as ready" for sex as she is, and usually take longer to get aroused.

"I've been dating younger guys because they can go and go and go like the Energizer bunny," she says. "We want the same things, so it's a good match."

One of her younger lovers (he was 23; she was 32) turned into a nine-month relationship, but Emily is currently not dating anyone seriously.

Like Anna, orgasms are pretty much guaranteed for this 30-something. Emily climaxes in every position, including with her partner on top, without additional clitoral stimulation.

"I think I have strong vaginal muscles," she says of her success rate. "Maybe because I would squat over the toilets in junior high and high school trying to pee in a straight line. I must have been so bored in school. I did it for years until I finally got tired of trying to control it. I'd even stop and try to hold it. I was doing Kegel exercises and had no clue."

Dr. Whelihan notes that Kegel exercises primarily strengthen pelvic floor muscles to prevent urine loss, and won't specifically facilitate orgasm. "But the fact that she has good pelvic floor control may indicate she is blessed with a heightened awareness and sensitivity in that area. And remember, while the glans of the clitoris is a bit far away from the vaginal opening, the 'legs,' or corpora, of the clitoris extend down around both sides of the vulva under the labia majora, so the stretch and stimulation there might be enough to help her reach climax with the man on top."

Emily says she's done no experimentation with girls, no role-playing and no anal sex. She does enjoy soft-core porn.

"That gets me kind of going, but I don't find heterosexual porn arousing," she clarifies. She enjoys gay porn, which she has watched with gay friends, because "the guys are so beautiful and their bodies are so hard."

By contrast, she dislikes "the money shots in heterosexual porn. I do not like seeing the vagina. The vagina disgusts . . . which is why I never experimented with girls, I guess."

An over-exuberant masturbatory experience at the age of 16 caused Emily to fear she had "rubbed off" her clitoris, and led to a months-long period when she refused to wash or otherwise care for her vagina. A later incident of a tampon becoming caught on her hymen (resulting in a hymenotomy), solidified Emily's hatred—her word—of her vagina.

Today, she still prefers not to look at vaginas, although she's willing to kiss a partner after he's gone down on her: "I don't really like to, but I have," she says.

"This comes up more than you might expect," says Dr. Whelihan. "Some women tell me this is a huge turnoff, but my response to them is a reminder that their juices should generally have a neutral taste and certainly not be unpleasant. In fact, a willingness to taste yourself indicates a confident and uninhibited appreciation of sex."

For Emily, each sexual encounter is its own reward.

"Why do it if it's not good?" she asks. "I know women who can't have orgasms, so they just do it to please their partners. If I'm not in the mood, I don't want to be touched. I don't even want to be kissed. I got to that point with my boyfriend in college. I still loved him, but I didn't want penetration. It was a big problem in our relationship; I think I was depressed. But that [period of disinterest in sex] was before my thirties. Now I think I could be talked into it."

PEAK? WHAT PEAK?

Charlie, a happily married mother of two, has experienced her thirties in a very different way; in fact, she answered the question about the biggest lie she'd been told about sex by saying, "That I'd hit my sexual peak in my thirties.

"My husband kept saying, 'When you hit your thirties, it'll be great,'" she says, but that hasn't been her experience.

"I don't know where I've come up with this discomfort about being sexual. I think I'm almost embarrassed to be sexual—even with my husband. I don't like to come to him [and ask for sex]. I don't ever feel a desire for sex, but once I get going, I start to have the desire to have an orgasm or whatever. But then that's all I care about."

Isn't the lead-up fun?

"No," she says, with a wince and a shrug. "And I don't know if I remember a time that it was fun."

Nevertheless, Charlie wrote in her survey that she's having the best sex of her life now, with her husband of 13 years, "because he cares to try; but I still don't like 'sex'; I just like the orgasm."

Dr. Whelihan notes that women are indeed often sexually neutral at any given time, whereas men have a more consistent sense of arousal due to their higher testosterone levels. Men must coax a woman from sexual neutrality to begin the process of arousal and desire in their partner.

"Don't mistake sexual neutrality as a lack of interest," says the doctor. "It's a natural state that just needs a partner's prompting. I advise women who aren't in the mood for sex not to say no to a request, but to say, 'I don't know; try to convince me.' That response encourages a man to kick up his game and remember his tricks of seduction, which will oftentimes be just the thing it takes to get her in the mood."

Charlie observes that her sex life has definitely improved as she and her husband have matured.

"We're more free with each other. I hate to say I don't like sex; I'm not sure that's true. On our 10th anniversary [at a nice hotel for the weekend], we must have had sex 10 times in 24 hours. Mostly quickies . . . it was fun. I was so free. We were drinking a little bit, no kids, no responsibility. . . . we were dedicated to each other. I don't feel that freeness in my everyday life. It's hard to create those experiences, but I think they're important."

Charlie has sex with her husband two to three times a week and achieves orgasm about 25 percent of the time (which corresponds to the times he performs oral sex).

"He enjoys when I have an orgasm and he enjoys bringing me there. . . . I can sense the type of sex we're going to have [based on] where the kids are, what time of day it is. I'll be more willing to give in if I know he's going to try to bring me to orgasm."

Charlie, an attractive professional athlete who grew up in Los Angeles, had a stressful introduction to sexual intercourse. At 15, she said yes to her boyfriend of nine months, who was 17.

"I had put him off and he was very kind about that," she relates. "I felt I'd kept him off long enough. He wasn't saying, 'If you don't have sex with me, I'll leave you,' but I'd been saying I wasn't ready, which implied that someday I *would* be ready. It felt like I had to be ready at some point. And it was a disaster.

"He was very large. I didn't know it at the time, until I had further sexual partners. He was very large and long and it was painful. I was dry, and not into it; I had no natural fluids going on, and he was too young to think of extra lubricant. It's vivid in my mind; I kind of remember him going in and out, and my whole vagina and lips were going in and out. You're trying to bite your tongue, thinking, 'It's gotta be over soon, right?'"

She tried to make the best of it and "not ruin his experience." Unfortunately, when he pulled out, the condom had broken and Charlie panicked.

"At 15, when you finally let it go . . . well, I freaked out. I made him drive me home immediately. We stopped on the way home at a drugstore so I could read the back of a pregnancy test. I was just trying to get information . . . he was trying to calm me down."

The couple eventually tried sex again and Charlie says it was a much better experience. They stayed together for another year, though she never experienced orgasms with him.

In fact, orgasm has never been easy for Charlie, who counts 14 or 15 lovers.

"When I was younger, I tried to figure things out, like, 'How am I going to pull this off for the rest of my life and make this work?' Because I faked [orgasms] all the time, just to get it done. I wondered, 'Is it ever going to change, and is it going to work and I won't have to fake it?' Maybe I have an enlarged clitoral hood and I can't get stimulated because there's too much around it. I thought I'd maybe ask someone when I got older, go to someone when I got more comfortable [on the subject]."

For women of any age wondering the exact same thing as Charlie, Dr. Whelihan says clitoral dysfunction in an otherwise healthy woman is most often affiliated with anxiety, but can also be due to trauma from a bicycle seat or a balance beam.

She explains that the clitoris has a hood, much like foreskin on a penis. In the United States, circumcision removes boys' foreskins, but female circumcision is not practiced. (In some cultures, female circumcision is done without anesthesia and as part of a sometimes-disfiguring ritual.)

In her practice, the doctor occasionally sees cases where the hood of the clitoris gets inflamed. "A tight band of tissue prevents the clitoral head from 'popping through' when engorged during arousal," she says. "This is called phimosis, and it can be surgically treated by opening up this scar band and even removing some redundant clitoral hood tissue."

That's rare, however. Much more often, the doctor says she sees situations where the clitoris is "buried" by excessive fat deposits on the mons pubis and vulva, and does not externalize even with proper engorgement and stimulation. Though Charlie's athleticism keeps her lean, Dr. Whelihan notes that obesity is the number one cause of this condition, which is easily remedied by weight loss.

Other issues that can make it difficult for a woman to climax are a lack of blood flow or even damaged nerves in the clitoral area (a permanent problem). "This is often seen in diabetes cases and, again, is preventable in most cases with diet and exercise."

If physical issues are ruled out, treatment techniques mirror those for anxiety disorders. Breathing and relaxation techniques are prescribed, along with practices such as using a blindfold to block out distractions and narrow the patient's focus to just the sense of touch.

BORN AGAIN

Charlie never got around to asking an expert whether she has an oversize clitoral hood, but a particularly dismal experience in her early twenties with an insensitive man led to a change in her whole approach.

"I was engaged to a Russian man, but sex with him was awful. He was rude and aggressive. After I broke up with him, I vowed I'd never have sex again until I was married, because it was so empty. I was done. I was so over it. I had given myself up too many times. I thought, 'What have I done with this gift?' And this was *before* I became a Christian."

The disillusionment with men together with her experience of becoming a born-again Christian convinced Charlie to become celibate. Nine months later, she met Alex, her future husband, who also is a Christian and had been celibate for four years. They dated for a little over a year, and did not engage in intercourse until their wedding night.

"I just decided to wait till the right person came along, to trust that it'd work," Charlie explains. "People said, 'What if he's big or small or he's not a good lover or whatever?' But I thought if two people love each other and have good communication, there's got to be a way to make it work. I believed in that."

The couple did have oral sex during their engagement, and Charlie experienced her first orgasms during this time as well, through manual stimulation from her fiancé.

To date, she's had only a few orgasms during penetration, and always when she's on top. Lately, her quickest route to orgasm (although they engage rarely) is the 69 position. Charlie says giving him oral sex arouses her and "everything is happening quickly."

She's not a fan of anal sex, however, naming it the one thing in regard to sex she wishes her partner would not attempt.

"One guy tried and failed," she recalls, and her husband used to playfully attempt to arouse her interest.

"He'd say there shouldn't be any place on my body he can't touch." But Charlie hasn't taken the bait.

ANAL TALK

Both Mickey and Emily share Charlie's view of anal sex. In fact, it's the most common response for 30-something women overall (with 15.2 percent) as the one thing they wish their partner would not do in regard to sex. (In second place, with 13 percent, was rushing to intercourse.)

"No guy has ever asked me to," Emily shares. "I've had people put their fingers up there, but I don't like it. I have IBS [irritable bowel syndrome], so I have diarrhea a lot . . . daily. There's always something coming out, so if something's going in, it makes it feel like something's going to come out."

Nevertheless, anal sex isn't something she's vetoed; she'd be willing to try it with someone she trusts. "And I'd have to be liquored up," she adds.

"I remember some friends in high school who had anal sex. One girl said as long as she was being fingered while it was happening she was okay."

Mickey says her ex-husband, Frank, used to ask for anal sex and "I said no, no, no. I used to play around and say, 'We can do it for our 80th anniversary.' I never said yes. My new boyfriend doesn't ask for that. He's very compassionate and caring. I'm sure some women like it, but he doesn't even ask, because he knows that I wouldn't want that."

Cyndi loves it, though. Her first partner was careful and she trusted him.

"He did the whole easing in, lubing up," she says. "He was very good about getting it in, and once it was in, I really liked it. I kept asking for it because I liked it so much. Once he said, 'What do you want for your birthday?' I said, 'Anal sex in the morning.' He said he felt like it was his birthday!"

But one of the girls she partnered with later didn't share

her enthusiasm.

"She didn't want me going near her butthole," Cyndi recalls, laughing. "She was one of those germophobes; she said, 'It's dirty in there.' She'd be afraid I would touch her vagina afterward, which is valid and all, but she was just über-cautious. We just didn't work. I'd keep trying to slip my hands in places and she didn't like it. I say, 'Those holes are there for a reason!' I couldn't get her to do it very often but I did try. I'm a little pushy." She grins.

THE CORE OF DESIRE

Our single and married interviewees diverge a bit on the question of what stimulates their desire. Since she shares a home with her boyfriend and is in a monogamous relationship, Mickey's views about desire align with those in the married group.

"Knowing I am truly loved and not just wanted sexually" makes Mickey willing to engage in intimacy. "When I am shown affection and shown how special I am, that makes me have the desire to be close and return appreciation."

"Kindness, humor, sometimes gentle caresses," says Anna, when asked what stimulates her desire.

But answers from single women sound different: "Verbal foreplay," is cited by Emily, who adds, "Alcohol definitely blocks the inhibitions." Cyndi relishes toys, porn and experimentation.

Which isn't to say there are not similarities between the single and married groups. Porn is popular across the aisle, with two-thirds of our interviewees mentioning it as at least an occasional turn-on. Worth noting is that most of those women did *not* include porn on their surveys to answer the question about what stimulates their desire. It was only during the in-depth interviews that this partiality was teased out, meaning there could be an issue of underreporting for the entire decade, where only 5 percent mentioned porn as a turn-on.

Case in point: Charlie's husband doesn't know she is titillated by porn. "I don't watch it on purpose," she says, "but if I see it when the guys are over and they're looking at a video, which is rare, it triggers something. I don't know how to describe it; I feel a change; blood starts flowing."

Another similarity for each interviewee in this decade is that—long before taking our survey—each woman had clearly given quite a bit of thought to her desires, her satisfaction and the quality of her sex life. Evidence of this degree of interest in sexuality isn't readily observed in the seventies, eighties and nineties decades, perhaps since society encouraged women of that era to channel their energies toward children and husbands, rather than dwelling on such personal needs.

With anywhere from 13 to 18 years of sexual activity under their belts (pun intended), our 30-something interviewees are nevertheless able to articulate how their desire has evolved during that relatively short time. And their answers are revealing.

Emily, as she noted earlier, yearns for sex in a way that is new since she entered her thirties. Tonya says her sex drive has diminished because her husband tells her no so often, and her heart longs for a female lover anyway.

But even in her lust for women, Tonya's process of sexual attraction has undergone a change.

"When I was younger, it was all physical," she says. "Now I desire a certain woman I'm close to who reciprocates the desire. There has to be an intellectual or spiritual connection before I feel desire. I don't just look at a woman and think, 'Wow, I'd like to sleep with her.' There has to be a connection. With us, it's holding hands, kissing, talking, her touching me. Something it's something as small as her putting her hand on my leg."

For Anna, trust has been the defining factor in the evolution of her desire, allowing her to become progressively more experimental, trying out spanking, anal sex, porn and more with her husband.

Charlie, too, is able to articulate precisely how her desire has evolved.

"Being monogamous, I've become less concerned with whether someone's going to approve [of] or like me because of sex," she says. "I think that was a huge factor in my development; sex was all about being accepted. I didn't want to be known as promiscuous, but I wanted guys to talk about me. Not necessarily that I was good in bed, but I wanted to be wanted by men. I knew my mom being nonsexual made my dad leave—and so I felt I had to learn how to make love. It wasn't until later on in my relationships that [the emphasis] would turn back toward me and I would concentrate on what *I* thought about sex, what *I* liked about it, what *I* wanted to get from it."

Mickey, our divorcée, said having a partner with a sex drive that matches hers has been a huge relief.

"I actually look forward to it at times; I desire the closeness, because I have that type of relationship where both of us want to be together," she says. "There's no guilt. And I don't feel like I'm just doing it, because my boyfriend never pressures me. Our sex drives are fairly equal, so that makes us compatible. My ex was off the charts; he wanted it every day. I always knew, if two or three days had gone by, he'd want it that night. Now if we go to the gym and we're tired, we just say so and we wait till the next night. Our sex drives are much more equal."

Although she and her boyfriend have sex once or twice a week now, Mickey says in the beginning it was more often.

"But you can't keep that up," she states. "I'd think, 'I can't wait to see him tonight,' and we'd have sex five days a week. It was a short period, but it was great. I finally felt at age 34 I was feeling what other women had felt, that attraction."

Of all our interviewees, perhaps Cyndi has undergone the most significant evolution in her sexual desire, since it has developed to include both sexes.

"I'm not writing men off," she says. "People ask if I'm lesbian now. No. I just want to find someone I can get along with that I enjoy being with. They ask, 'Which way do you lean; who do you think you'll end up with?' I have no clue. I really don't know. I just know I've increased my chance of meeting that person by a hundred percent because I can do man or woman. People want to label people too much. I'm like, why? All this classification stuff . . . I say don't box me in."

As for her sex drive, Cyndi describes it as being on a continual incline.

"It's been ramping up. As long as I've been having sex, I've always had a very strong sexual desire. It's just gotten stronger. I allow myself to explore and that makes my desire greater.

"As for the future, I don't know. There are so many things I want to try. My mind is like, 'What can I do next?' I think if you allow yourself to have that sex drive, then it'll be there."

The colorful interviews with women from this eventful decade show that they understand both the psychological mechanisms of desire as well as the physical processes that enable them to achieve satisfying sexual encounters. We found women in their teens and twenties were more often familiar with only physical attraction and the resulting arousal.

So are the thirties truly the period of a woman's sexual peak? With no hard scientific evidence to support what is basically an urban legend, it's impossible to say. But our evidence shows that certainly 30-something women are confident in their own understanding of sexual desire, how it pertains to their relationships and the importance of both to their overall quality of life.

DECADES OF DESIRE:
THE FORTIES

As a whole, the spokeswomen for the forties decade show themselves to be a startlingly communicative group. One tells of her short career—two to three years—as a high-priced call girl; another reveals halfway through our interview that she was molested at the age of 9 by her father; another confides that she has never experienced an orgasm, and yet another shares intimate smartphone pictures of her with her lover.

Exactly 300 women in their forties filled out our survey on desire, making this decade the largest in our sampling. The fifties were a close second, with just 11 fewer representatives. The large numbers are no surprise, since gynecological checkups are of prime importance for women in both age groups.

Coincidentally, our in-depth interviews captured women in the second half of the forties, with all respondents born between 1965 and 1970. Each woman joined the world when American sexual mores were undergoing the most substantial face-lift in a century, so most escaped the rigorous behavior restrictions of previous generations. Nevertheless, the phrase "I was a good girl" pops up repeatedly during interviews with women in this age group. Though born in an era of sexual experimentation, they are deeply sensitive to the culture's continued classification of a "bad girl."

Not only do forties women open up during interviews about their desires and preferences, but at this age they've also become adept at letting their partners know their hearts' desires. "Here's what I like," is a frequent conversation starter in the bedroom—and several forties women say they're thrilled with the resultant intimacy.

In some cases, however, getting to "here's what I like" took time. With encouragement from a marriage counselor, Linda, a 46-year-old mother of two, was eventually able to share what "worked" for her sexually with her husband, though it took years of togetherness for her to be comfortable enough to do so.

"When I first told him, I think I showed him and did it while he was inside me," says Linda, who's been married 23 years. "I call it 'lazy sex'; it's like spoon sex, where I have my hand free and available to rub my clitoris. Opening up like that to someone and making myself vulnerable turned me on and made me enjoy it thoroughly."

Her husband's acceptance, several years into their marriage, was a milestone for Linda, who had not achieved orgasm with previous partners.

"Unless you're open about sex and what you like having done—which I wasn't with him at first; maybe I was scared of being hurt—you're not able to enjoy it thoroughly. Some women may be uninhibited and able to say right away what they like or don't, but that wasn't me."

Despite the relatively enlightened era in which she was raised, Linda's initial inability to express her needs may have had to do with parents who shamed her when they caught her in youthful exploration.

"I felt sexual from a very young age—like 5 or 6. I knew how to give myself an orgasm at that young age. I just put my hands between my legs and started rubbing. I knew it felt good and so I did it. But I remember getting caught by my parents a couple of times and they told me it was bad. So I got the impression it wasn't good to have orgasms. But I still did it because it felt good."

During the early years of her marriage, Linda sometimes masturbated beside her husband when he'd fallen asleep after sex that hadn't been fulfilling for her.

"I did feel sneaky about [the masturbation], but it was part of the excitement," she says, noting that she didn't fake orgasms. "This was before I was honest and told him that I *could* have an orgasm and this is how. The marriage counselor opened us up so we could communicate about sex."

A WHOLE LOT OF SHAKING (BUT NO FAKING) GOING ON

Though their frequency of orgasm varies from never to 100 percent of the time, no interviewee in this decade is currently faking it to satisfy a partner or boost his ego. A few said they did so as young women, but no more.

Carmen, who was raised in a conservative Catholic Hispanic family, has sex two or three times a week with her husband of 24 years, and is not hiding from him the fact that she never orgasms.

"I think I faked it a couple times when we were first married," she says. "He wanted me to orgasm so much and he would try so hard. But we've discussed that it's okay if I don't. As long as he's happy, I'm happy."

As Carmen outlines the early days of their courting—the

couple dated for 2½ years before marrying—her maidenly modesty is apparent.

"I was very inexperienced; I was a good girl," she says. "I remember him pushing the envelope with me. I was 18 and he couldn't even cop a feel of my breast. He was my first kiss too. That first kiss was wonderful. I'd never been kissed like that. I'd never allowed it. He was my first everything."

Carmen says she's deeply satisfied with her marriage, but that's not to say she wouldn't welcome a change in her sex life.

"I do want to learn to get over this orgasm hang-up so I can be more sexually fulfilled in my older years, when the kids are gone and we don't have to worry who's listening or if someone's going to walk in on us. But the more I harp on it, the more out of reach it is. Sometimes when we're having sex I think, 'I'm not going to think about it,' and then I end up the whole time thinking, 'I'm not going to think about it!'"

The couple has experimented with toys in their quest for her elusive orgasm, but the happily married Carmen doesn't allow this issue to define her relationship.

"We have a great connection," she says. "He's a great guy. When I met him, I knew he was the one. [Now] I have more desire for an intimate relationship, rather than sex. We can lie in bed and laugh and talk for hours. In the car, we talk and talk and laugh. I know couples who go out together and don't have 10 words to say, but we are so loving. I can't imagine my life without him.

"Even though I can't reach orgasm with my husband, I want to be with him; I want to satisfy him, and I'm hoping that for me one day I can reach orgasm. I think if I can do that, he's going to be so happy that finally we were able to solve this thing that we've had between us for 20 something years."

Bonnie, 48, is another woman who's honest with her husband about when she does or doesn't have orgasms. The native Floridian with shoulder-length hair and an open, freckled face says her percentage of reaching orgasm with her second husband hovers around 50 percent.

"When we first got together, it was less," says this full-time student who worked in utility construction for 30 years. "And he would like me to have an orgasm every time. I think I've finally made him realize I don't have to have an orgasm to feel good. Sometimes I do, but sometimes I'm like, 'No, I'm good.' We've been together long enough that he can say, 'I came. I know you want to come, so let's make you come.'"

Bonnie's husband knows how to give her orgasms with his hand or toys, but he also loves it if she does it herself, although sometimes this embarrasses her.

"I don't want the lights on or to be on display," she explains, noting that talking during sex still doesn't come easily for her. Cuddling and sharing what's going on is fine, "but don't watch me like I'm on a movie screen."

LADIES LIVING LARGE

Though we just met a pair of women still working toward the full expression of their sexuality, the majority of our forties interviewees claim very high percentages of achieving orgasm— along with an anything-that-works policy in the bedroom.

So let's meet these ladies.

Heather, a zaftig blonde and our aforementioned call girl, was 21 the first time she had sex, and is another woman who uses the phrase "I was a good girl" to describe herself.

"I grew up in a neighborhood [in Miami] where at 16 we were still kids; we weren't adults. None of my friends had sex in their teens in the group I grew up with. There was Spin the Bottle, sure, and we might kiss or someone might touch your breast, but that was *huge*."

Throughout her teens, Heather was overweight, shy and not much interested in boys or sex. She assumed she would wait until she was married to lose her virginity.

But at 21, while on a date with a male friend, she changed her mind.

"He was a similar age, but it wasn't his first time," she recalls. "I didn't even know what to do; I was such a sheltered child. But I was curious."

She doesn't remember either liking or disliking the experience, and desire didn't enter into the equation, but she found sex interesting and wanted to try it again. Before long, she experimented with a second partner, and then retreated from sex altogether for a time.

"I was appalled at having been with two people, when I was so sure I'd wait till marriage. I felt it wasn't right, so I stopped for a few years. I wasn't ready, I guess."

In her late 20s, aerobic exercise led to a drastic body change for Heather and she became a part-time instructor in Los Angeles. She began dating again and even lived with a couple of boyfriends. She was in her thirties when her full-time job as a legal secretary ended, and that's when—seemingly more or less on a whim—she hit upon the idea of turning tricks.

"It wasn't walking on the street," she clarifies. "I would never do that, ever. I worked for a high-end escort service. It's funny, because I was the most wholesome girl you could imagine. It's so unlike me to do that. But I majored in theater in college, and it was basically just putting on an act. It was a job. I never thought of it as anything else. It wasn't sex; it was a job."

Nevertheless, Heather says that on her first time out she had to stop to throw up.

The work—which she calls a victimless crime that shouldn't be illegal—supported her for a couple of years and she earned enough money for plastic surgery on her breasts and buttocks. "After I lost all the weight I got everything lifted," she reports. "I made a ton of money. It was $300 or $400 a pop, and I could be in and out in 15 minutes—and do more than one in a night. I can't even tell you how many guys: maybe over 500 during those years. I don't count them."

Heather, now 50, says she never climaxed on the job ("I'd fake it just to get out of there"). In her personal life, however, she experiences orgasm with all her sexual encounters, and there have been many, since after her call girl days she spent years "in the lifestyle," meaning she was part of a swinger culture.

"There's no point in faking it," she says regarding bedroom bliss. "If it's not working, I'll say, 'Hey, let's try this,' so that we can eventually get there. But it doesn't necessarily happen right away."

Sassy, a delicate, 49-year-old blonde with two grown children and an airy, colorfully decorated home in South Florida, echoes Heather's sentiments. She too finds orgasms achievable with every encounter, but the process does take some time.

"I don't have orgasms easily," she relates. "It takes me a while. If he's in my ass, I can orgasm with clitoral stimulation [using her fingers], but I think my favorite way is with him on top but sort of on the side."

Her boyfriend, a man 12 years her junior who's been a calendar model, is by far her favorite of her five lovers.

"We usually have sex for two hours, and sometimes I'll have three orgasms. But they're so strong it's usually hard to have another. He likes to go down on me and try to eat me after I orgasm, but I'm so sensitive it hurts."

She notes she hasn't yet experienced an orgasm from her boyfriend performing oral sex, and since this is a bit unusual, we'll use it as a segue into a quick look at exactly how popular oral sex is—*very!*—for all women and, more important, how crucial clitoral stimulation is.

ORAL SEX: A BIG WINNER

Our 300-strong forties decade is fairly representational of all survey respondents on this acclaimed subject. When asked for their quickest route to orgasm, 22 percent in this decade name oral sex; another 22 percent say clitoral stimulation without distinguishing what type. A vibrator to the clitoris is the answer for another 11 percent of women in this decade, and yet another 28 percent are split between manual stimulation and masturbation.

So, if you're keeping count, that means 83 percent of women this age don't even *mention* penetration when they reveal their path to orgasm. (This holds true for all ages, yet still manages to surprise men, 35 years after Shere Hite set the record straight in *The Hite Report on Female Sexuality, 1976*.)

For their quickest route, the *only* orgasmic position named by women more than a handful of times is "me on top." Not coincidentally, this position stimulates a woman's clitoris through friction with her partner's pubic bone during penetration. Accordingly, 9 percent of women name this as their quickest route.

That brings the total to 92 percent of women who directly or indirectly require clitoral stimulation for orgasm. The remaining 8 percent of 40-something women answer this survey question by naming a dozen or so less-traveled paths to orgasm. Answers include G-spot stimulation, extended foreplay, slow penetration, gentle play with nipples, fantasy thoughts, deep penetration, feeling in control and more.

WHAT'S YOUR QUICKEST ROUTE TO ORGASM?

	ORAL SEX	CLITORAL STIMULATION (non-specific)*	TOTAL
Teens	14.8%	11.1%	25.9%
20s	20.7%	17.9%	38.6%
30s	28.5%	13.9%	42.4%
40s	21.7%	11.7%	33.3%
50s	21.5%	13.1%	34.6%
60s	21.2%	18.7%	39.9%
70s	20.3%	19.5%	39.8%
80s	3.8%	15.4%	19.2%
90s	0.0%	36.4%	36.4%

*This table targets oral sex, and doesn't include answers that specifically named masturbation or vibrator use as the quickest route to orgasm.

EXCEPTIONS TO EVERY RULE

Numbers don't lie, and our survey shows oral sex is a favorite for women of all ages, but our actual face-to-face interviewees in this decade don't all happen to be fans. In fact, they are split 50-50 on its charms.

Bonnie, who counts 28 or 29 lovers, remembers only one time when she had an orgasm from oral sex.

"I thinks it's because he sucked a lot," she speculates, "instead of [treating it] like it's a salt lick."

She's been married and monogamous for 10 years now; she and husband John have one son.

"I've been told I taste good—by more than one guy. Many,

in fact," she says a bit shyly. "My husband likes the way I taste. If he goes down on me, yes, it's pleasurable, but it's more of a desire thing, you know? Being wanted that way. He loves it."

But she doesn't come.

"It's not unpleasant," she clarifies. "It's not repulsive by any means. It's nice; it's comforting. I just figure, 'I'm not going to get off on it, but let's have fun.' I say go for it."

Linda, our fan of "spoon sex," says it's been years since her husband performed oral sex on her.

"I'd rather just use the vibrator. I'm sure he's okay with that. I sweat between the crack of my legs and sometimes it's not a pleasant environment. I don't know if that's an age thing or if it's just me, but that's one of my inhibitions, wanting to feel clean and smell clean before we have sex."

Linda's overall opinion of oral sex: "It's not the same as a vibrator; what can I say?"

Sage, a 47-year-old executive assistant, also is lukewarm on the subject.

"It's not my top thing," she says. "I prefer penetration. I'll say, 'I want to feel you inside me.'" She notes that she can get the same stimulation through tilting her pelvis during rear-entry sex, assuring that—during deep penetration—the shaft of his penis creates clitoral stimulation [through stretching].

But does she *like* oral sex?

"I don't find it necessary," she answers.

Carmen, who gives her husband blow jobs because she knows he enjoys them, also doesn't care to be on the receiving end. Oral sex makes her feel uncomfortable and it's been several years since her husband tried.

"I've tolerated it," she says. "But usually I go, 'I have to shower; I have to shave,' and tell him why it can't be today.

[Maybe] I feel unclean, even though he says he likes the way it looks, he likes the way it smells."

Amy, a 48-year-old lesbian in a long-term relationship, and a fan of oral sex, also brought up the importance of personal hygiene.

"Things that are natural can be a turnoff," she says with a shrug, specifically mentioning bad breath, belching and farting. "When you're so comfortable with someone that you can walk into the bathroom and there they are on the toilet . . . and shortly after they want to have sex . . . well, now I've got the visual image of you taking a crap," she says.

TOO MUCH, TOO LITTLE, JUST ENOUGH?

Amy, who had sex with her first girlfriend in ninth grade, says she does not have a high sex drive, and that her partner, Barb, possesses a more active libido. At first the couple made love every day; now it's once or twice a month.

But is that unusual?

In her lectures on sexual function, Dr. Mo enjoys educating the public on just how broad a spectrum the word *normal* encompasses when it comes to frequency of sex. We've touched on this before, but it's worth restating.

"Someone with an average sex drive has sex once a week, someone with a low sex drive wants sex once a month, and someone with a high sex drive wants sex once a day—and *all* of those degrees of sex drive are normal," stresses Dr. Whelihan.

Proving her case, we met two other forties women who report numbers close to Amy's for frequency of sex: Linda says she and her husband make love one to three times a month; Bonnie reports two or three times monthly.

Sassy and her younger lover started out having sex twice

a day, four days a week when they first got together, but busy schedules now have them at about twice weekly. (She believes that number would increase if he were to move in.) Heather, who is in a six-year relationship, says they had sex three times a day in the beginning; now they have sex once or twice a week. Nonorgasmic Carmen has sex with her husband two to three times a week, and Sage, who's married to her second husband, reports the highest consistent number of women in this decade: three to five times a week (after 14 years of marriage).

Gabriella, whose father raped her, had sex as infrequently as possible with her husband of 13 years. They divorced eight years ago and she's had no lovers since.

But, of course, frequency is only one piece of the picture, so let's fill in satisfaction numbers for the rest of our interviewees. Heather claims 100 percent satisfaction, Carmen is at zero and Bonnie estimates she climaxes 50 percent of the time. Sassy reports she's also at 100 percent, while Amy and Linda estimate 95 percent. Gabriella, whose only lover was her husband, began having orgasms after several years of marriage, and reports that she climaxed only when they had oral sex, which was about 10 percent of the time. Sage says her number is 75 percent.

"In general, women who can achieve orgasm more than 75 percent of the time have no underlying issues," notes Dr. Whelihan. "It's simply that life stresses can occasionally inject themselves into the encounter and interfere with her ability to relax and achieve orgasm. Anyone at that percentage is functioning at a high level."

The doctor says it's worth noting that women who can reach orgasm during sex are more likely to approach the next encounter with enthusiasm, because they anticipate a pleasurable outcome.

However, orgasm isn't a requirement for sex to be considered satisfactory. Most women are not going to climax with every single intimate encounter, but that doesn't mean there's no pleasure in the act.

"On the other hand, women who rarely or never climax—either because their partner lacks the skills to help them or because the woman has no expectation of achieving climax—are much less likely to initiate sex," she says. "Additionally, this is the age group where erectile dysfunction begins to surface because of medical problems in men, so those difficulties may lead to more stress and less satisfaction for both partners."

While climaxing is a sure-fire way to rate a sexual encounter as a success, our interviewees validate Dr. Whelihan's statement that satisfying sex can occur without an orgasm. (Though men don't tend to agree.)

Bonnie, who climaxes half the time, says the intimacy of sex is sometimes enough.

"Guys don't understand that. For them it's all or nothing," she says. "They don't get it. They can't just feel good by having a hard-on and it goes away. It *must* end in orgasm. But women, the desire and intimacy are a big part of it . . . the closeness and feeling connected to that person.

"I wouldn't have sex with someone just because they were attractive; it would only be with someone I wanted a commitment with," she continues. "If you are having sex with too many people you're not interested in having a relationship with, you may lose that ability to connect. [Sex] shouldn't be like going out to get a massage. It should be special."

Bonnie sees a clear difference between sex and making love.

"Sex can be with anyone or anything: It's just a physical activity that is pleasurable for your body. But making love has the intimacy of touch, caress, looking into somebody's eyes and feeling this is somebody you want to be with over time. It's not just, 'Thanks. Good-bye.'"

Ask Bonnie what sustains sexual desire over the long haul, and her deep connection to her husband is apparent; she acknowledges both the emotional and purely physical aspects of their relationship.

"I can't think of being with anyone else; I don't want to be. And I feel confident that he's feeling the same way about me. *This* is the person I make love to. Even if it is [an occasion] when I just want sex, this is the person I turn to. He understands that, 'Yeah, I want to get off.'"

WHAT STIMULATES DESIRE, VERSUS WHAT SUSTAINS IT

Our survey canvasses women on what stimulates their desire, but it is the in-depth interviews that plumb the more ideological question of what sustains that desire. There's usually a sharp contrast in how the forties ladies respond to these two questions.

Bonnie, who articulately addresses the "sustain" question in the previous section, says her desire is generally stimulated by circumstances, such as her kids being asleep, the bed being cleaned off and her husband not being asleep in front of the TV or computer. It also helps if *she's* not half-asleep.

Once those conditions are right, Bonnie responds to her husband holding her tight, kissing her neck, maybe grabbing her behind while he's holding her . . . "*desiring* me, just being desired," she says.

Linda and Sage, who are also each married with children, give answers that echo Bonnie's.

"To begin with, I need total relaxation," says Linda, "a free and clear mind without worries, knowing I don't have to work, clean, [deal with] kids. I can't be angry or mad at my husband or thinking about work weighing me down. Swimming naked in the hot tub helps, knowing someone might catch us."

Sage says she favors a mental trifecta to stimulate her desire: No stress, a little romance and the desire to connect. Plus some alcohol!

"Stress is such a part of everyone's lives," she says. "A few drinks help iron out the wrinkles that are always there. This is truer with a long-term partner because you have the shared stresses of bills, kids, maybe a business together, et cetera. Sometimes it's tough to separate that aspect of the relationship and just be in the moment and enjoy the physicality. It's hard to shut off that you're three days late on the water bill or the kid just brought home an F.

"I can see why role-playing can be such a turn-on," Sage concludes. "I can see why you want to get away from the whole realistic relationship that you have. Reality is not an aphrodisiac."

But to *sustain* desire, Sage believes trust is key.

"For me personally, it's so mental. There has to be a level of trust, which I have with my partner now. You must have the utmost trust. Once that's broken, I start to shut down emotionally and am not interested in a sexual relationship with the individual. It takes a lot for me to lose trust; little things don't bother me so much. But for me, in a monogamous relationship, him breaking those vows would make me lose trust."

Linda's answer for what sustains desire is short and sweet: "Obviously, a good, honest relationship that can make you forget momentarily about the everyday stress."

Amy agrees with Sage on what sustains desire: "The first

thing that comes to mind is you have to love someone and trust them. Intimacy is like trust; it's such a fragile thing. Once it's broken, it's done. You're baring yourself, your soul; you're naked before your partner."

Her answer for what stimulates her desire is, "Smell, a great smile and beautiful eyes."

Carmen says "holding hands, romance, talking and spending time alone" stimulate her desire, but she has trouble articulating what sustains desire, because that's been an uphill battle her whole life.

"When we were younger it was the attraction to each other that we couldn't get enough of. Now that we're older, it's more intimate to me. I love him so much that I don't mind having sex. I do it because I know he wants it and it makes him happy. I don't have that passion anymore. I wish I did. But I still want to satisfy him. That's why we have sex frequently. I don't like saying no."

Heather is on the other end of the spectrum from Carmen, saying her desire for sex has increased as she's aged.

"There's a difference between having sex in your twenties and having sex in your forties. In your forties you're horny all the time. It's terrible; it never stops. [For me] it started in my mid-thirties and hasn't stopped."

Heather lists touch, closeness, imagination, thoughts and kisses as stimulants to her desire. To keep the fires alive, she too references the mental component: "I would think being mutually respectful of each other and loving each other sustains the desire. If you start growing apart mentally you're not going to be so interested in [sex]."

Sassy's answers for the two questions both contain the word *chemistry*. On her survey, she wrote that what stimulates her desire is "a hot man (my boyfriend) kissing me; holding hands because I'm attracted to him; it stimulates me to want more; chemistry; sends shivers through me and I get wet."

Sustaining desire, she says, requires "chemistry and knowing your partner and their needs. And them knowing your needs." She notes that her second husband was selfish and not affectionate. "I need to feel special and loved and wanted and desired, and he didn't give me that. And I had no sexual desire for him. None."

THE WIDER VIEW

Though not surveyed on what sustains desire, the larger group of 40-somethings had plenty to say about what stimulates it.

Like most decades, these women name kissing as the number one stimulant: 16 percent choose it. (For an open-ended question, with infinite responses possible, that's a very high number.) No other answer garners more than 8 percent of the total, but four answers did hit that percentage: slow foreplay, being in love (or feeling loved), wine, and some form of touching.

In smaller numbers, the other half of women in this decade name such things as cuddling, the smell of a man's cologne, porn, thoughts of a past lover, getting away for the weekend, being listened to, their partner's good looks, breast stimulation, a sexy look from their partner and quite a few other stimulants.

When we ask 40-something women to pinpoint the best sex of their life, 13.5 percent say they are still waiting for it, and 14 percent say it was in their thirties. But the most popular answer (16.5 percent) is now, in their forties.

BEST SEX IS "RIGHT NOW" BY DECADE

Teens	0%	(most answered they were still waiting for it)
20s	4.8%	(34% answered "with the love of my life"; 24% were still waiting)
30s	26%	
40s	15.5%	
50s	13%	
60s	10%	
70s	2%	
80s	7%	

This table reflects a Bell curve until the eighties, a decade when the percentage of satisfaction jumps, perhaps reflecting the women's delight and gratitude to be having a still-active sex life in this phase of their lives.

In general, 40-something women showed approval for their mates, making "nothing, he's great," the number one answer (with 25 percent) to the question, "What is the one thing you wish your partner would not do in regard to sex?" This seems like a large number of women who don't even occasionally wish their partner would slow down or perhaps be a bit more adventuresome or maybe talk less or any of the myriad suggestions survey takers name.

Perhaps the contentment of 40-something women stems from the fact that they've learned to speak up in bed and ask for what they want. Or maybe women this age are simply less picky, and truly satisfied with reality.

MOST COMMON COMPLAINTS
OF 40-SOMETHINGS

RUSHING TO INTERCOURSE	11.6%
TOO MUCH TALK/DIRTY TALK	11.6%
ATTEMPTS AT ANAL	10.0%
INSENSITIVITY	9.5%
SPANKING	5.0%

Those who did pick a complaint name spanking; attempts to have anal sex; being insensitive to her needs; rushing to intercourse; and either talking dirty or just talking too much. Laziness, poor hygiene and using fingers too roughly are mentioned less frequently, along with "waking me up for sex," biting nipples and "pushing on my head during oral sex."

Survey-wide, almost 12 percent of women name anal sex as their least-favorite bedroom scenario, so interviewees are asked to elaborate.

Our 40-somethings show a split in their interest, with Sassy, Linda and Bonnie giving it at least an occasional thumbs-up, while Gabriella, Carmen and Sage just say no. A quote from each camp should suffice to sum up the opposing viewpoints.

"That's an egress; entry will never happen," asserts Sage. "In the very beginning, [my husband] was adamant that he wanted to try everything. I was a good sport up until the head of his penis went in, and then there was this blinding, searing pain. I thought, 'This feels like childbirth. I no longer feel like having an orgasm or having sex with you.' I don't know who loves this, but it's not for me. Keep all penises, fingers and other objects away from the egress."

Bonnie, however, says anal sex is fine for "something differ-ent," but generally finds other variations work better.

"What you can do is use a vibrator in your butt and him inside your pussy," she shares. "And it will alter [the experience] so that when he's penetrating you, it pushes him in a different direction and directs him to my G-spot."

Bonnie says this enables her husband to become stimulated by the feel of the tickly vibrator, and can help make the mission-ary position more enjoyable for women.

"Because missionary for a woman is kind of ho-hum," she claims [to a chorus of "amen" from women everywhere]. "The vibrator pushes his penis more into the position as if he's enter-ing from behind," she explains. "It doesn't need to be fat at all," she says of the vibrator. "It should be more long than fat."

THE MORE, THE MERRIER

As long as the subject of adventurous sexual practices has come up, let's tour the topic of threesomes. No statistics can be pulled for our wider survey population, but since everything surfaces during in-depth interviews, it transpires that half of this decade's interviewees have taken part in a threesome. For Linda and Sage, it was a one-time-only event; Heather reports multiple incidences, and Sassy has participated in one threesome with two men and one with another woman and her lover.

Interestingly, none of the women had a burning desire for threesome sex prior to her experience. In several cases it hap-pened spontaneously and was accompanied by copious amounts of alcohol.

Sage, whose first marriage lasted seven years, says she tried group sex one time with her first husband, her best friend and the friend's husband.

"There was lots of alcohol involved," she recalls cheerily. "It started as a foursome, but it ended up just she and I, with them watching. It's not that I felt terrible, but it wasn't something I had any interest in pursuing. It's not a lifestyle that works for me necessarily."

After happily experimenting with between 20 and 30 partners in college ("I went wild! I was from a strict, Catholic home, so for me it was drugs, alcohol and men for sex on a regular basis. I'm sorry, a degree was secondary!"), Sage settled down and became monogamous with a fellow student, who later became husband number one.

"He was a raging alcoholic," she states, and the relationship ended a month after their son was born. "I realized you can choose crazy for yourself," she summarizes, "but it's beyond unfair to choose it for your kid." She packed up and left, and hasn't looked back—or tried a threesome since.

Linda also mentions a brief foray into group sex, which occurred when she and her husband lived in Ohio years ago. They became friendly with several couples, forming a group that drank shots and played a card game called Asshole after their kids went to sleep.

"There was one point where we were showing the tits," she recalls. "That took a lot of guts, but when you're drunk you lose your inhibitions. It was exciting, I guess. And in one instance, a guy whipped out his weenie and his wife sucked on it. So I did have the experience of seeing couples show their stuff in a drunken state."

During one of these gatherings, Linda and her husband retreated to the backyard to have sex, knowing their friends would try to watch in the dark. She found that exciting as well.

But her actual group sex experience wasn't that much fun.

"It was this one time with another couple; we were drunk and my husband actually had sex with the other woman. It kind of bothered me at the time. I sat on top of her husband . . . he was heavy. It didn't take long for him. I was uninhibited but not that into it. I was probably thinking [my husband] was having more fun with her than I was with him. She was skinny . . . and he wasn't the most attractive. I felt he was getting the better end of the deal."

Though she describes the incident as a part of her past, "just a drunken, stupid thing we all did," she and her husband do occasionally talk about the encounter to become stimulated.

"I think we both may have experienced jealousy," she says. "We got it out of our system, and discovered it's not really worth it. Anyway, we don't still drink like that. It was a little phase and it wound down."

Heather, whose time "in the lifestyle" in Los Angeles took away her reservations about group sex, has done threesomes and more.

"At one [swingers'] party, I had a small gang bang . . . five or six guys. That was pretty interesting. It seems a whole lifetime ago. Now my days are pretty boring, which I don't like."

Back then, whenever she participated in threesomes with a woman and a man, Heather let it be known that she wouldn't be touching the woman.

"Most people knew that I don't do women, so I didn't have to worry about that. I'm very straight."

Heather is currently in an unsatisfying relationship; at six years and counting, it's her longest. She's also having an affair with a married man she met about a year ago, and recently set up a threesome for him, but he backed out.

"Then he arranged a threesome on his boat with another

guy, because he thinks that's what I want, but I got shy that day for some reason," she admits. "I don't know why. I do get like that every so often."

Sassy, as mentioned before, has had experiences with both male and female additions during trysts with her lover. A widow at 22, who quickly remarried for stability, Sassy did not have an adventurous love life before Maurice.

"Now sex is like starring in our own porn movie," she enthuses.

However, venturing into new territory isn't risk-free.

"He gave me a threesome with a guy about four months ago—but it sucked," Sassy reports. "It was very disappointing. I had agreed to it way back when Maurice first asked, hoping he would get jealous. Anyway, we were at Maurice's house and his roommate was there. Maurice called him [into the bedroom] when we were naked and told him to take pictures. . . . He took pictures of me eating Maurice's ass. Then Maurice tells him to take off his clothes. He puts on a condom [and] I didn't want to touch it. I was touching rubber; there's nothing to touch. So I was touching his balls. Then Maurice tells him to fuck me. And he's inside me, fucking me, but I didn't feel it much . . . maybe he was small."

Despite her disappointment, Sassy reports that Maurice came quickly during the encounter and then had two more orgasms while his friend was "moaning and groaning" while inside her, presumably in delight.

"I really go out of my way to please [Maurice] and give him whatever he asks," she says. "I tell him, 'I loved my first husband, but it doesn't compare to what I feel for you.' Even just watching TV with him, I am so content, so happy. I love our sleepovers, with just him next to me. Sometimes I just stare at him. He's like this movie star; I can't get enough of him. Doing his laundry makes me happy. Doesn't that sound stupid? I love having it here, folding it. It makes me feel like he's here."

Her devotion led Sassy to consent to a second threesome, despite her reservations—this time with another woman.

"I didn't want to share him because I really, really love him and I knew it would hurt me," she says. When she broached her fears with Maurice, he reminded her of their three-year relationship by asking, "Who am I with?" And he reassured her, "It's just sex."

"I should get the fucking award for Best Girlfriend of the Year." Sassy laughs. "In his eyes, he thinks any girl would do this for him, but I tend to think not."

So a couple of months ago, she and Maurice went shopping for a strap-on to use in the threesome. Maurice insisted she try it on in the store, and despite her embarrassment, she eventually did. A purchase was made.

Sassy narrates the subsequent threesome encounter:

"She took off her clothes and was just waiting. I tried kissing her. I was sucking on her boobs and she wouldn't reciprocate. I don't know what I'm doing, but I'm trying to be a good sport. So I was masturbating her while he was fucking her. Or while he's fucking her from behind, I'm eating his ass. I'm trying to be a good sport, but I haven't done this before. '*You* want this fantasy; I'm trying to make it come true for you.' It's hard to have sex and talk at the same time. You have to think of these things . . . like I was pushing him into her harder or using the phone to take different-angle pictures of him inside of her so he has them to look back on. What girlfriend does this kind of thing?"

So I ask her: "What girlfriend does these things?"

"Someone who really loves this guy," she answers. "It's a woman who loves this man so much. . . . I keep telling him, 'I would do anything for you.'"

Back at the threesome, Sassy says it was time to do the strap-on.

"I straddle over the bed and put it in that way first. That wasn't doing it, so she lies down. I've never done this. . . . I'm inserting a cock inside her for the first time. I asked, 'Am I hurting you?' I put the vibration on, while he's taking photos and video. I'm kissing her. . . . I'm trying. He said afterward he had a feeling so incredible, like butterflies, when he watched me do that. He said he's never had anything like that feeling."

Though Maurice would like to repeat the experience, Sassy says she was a little bored and felt like a third wheel: "It was kind of hard to watch him make her come three times."

She concludes that threesomes aren't for everyone, because they can backfire.

"There can be issues of jealousy; the other women can be trying to steal your man. If I were being selfish, I wouldn't want to share him. [Threesomes] aren't something that's high on my list.

"But this is the kind of guy he is," she concludes philosophically. "He seems to need and want it. He's going to cheat on the side and I'd rather him do it with me. I think we're both kinky. Thinking of his explosion, his erection, that's what gets me excited."

Maurice is her fifth lover, and Sassy says that while in the past sex felt good and she wanted it, now it means much more. One of her recent strategies in the bedroom is to actually consider, "If I was a penis, what would I like?"

"I'm always trying to please him, to wow him, make him excited and happy. If he's happy, I'm happy. I try to put him first, and I didn't do that for the others."

WHAT'S YOUR NUMBER?

Unlike the 30-something women we interviewed, women in this decade do not exhibit regret or even conflicted feelings about the number of lovers they've taken throughout their lifetime. Twelve is their average, but it's not the number, it's the acceptance of it that is noticeable. Dr. Mo points to the sweet spot inhabited by these women, each of whom graduated from high school between 1983 and 1988.

"Not only do women in their forties have the luck of being raised when sexual liberation was the norm, but by this age they have also learned how to accept their body and understand what gives, or doesn't give them pleasure," says Dr. Mo. "They often feel empowered by their sexuality and their ability to control the outcome in the bedroom. It's a win-win for all parties."

The number of lovers for women in this decade range from one (for both Carmen and Gabriella) to approximately 800 (for Heather, if we include the 500 or so partners she serviced while working as a call girl). The other women vary from five (Sassy) to 29 (Bonnie). Linda counts eight and Amy claims a dozen.

By dropping Heather's unusually high total, we arrive at the aforementioned average of 12. For comparison, 30-somethings averaged 14 partners, and 50-something interviewees had 13. (In the fifties decade, one woman also had a high number of partners, probably more than 500, and she was dropped from that decade's average.)

Some 40-somethings began sexual activity fairly early. Keeping in mind that—survey-wide—13 is the youngest age *anyone* lists for a first-time (consensual) sexual encounter, we interviewed four women (Amy, Sassy, Linda and Sage) in this decade who started at age 14, and another who started at 15 (Bonnie).

But delayed starts for other interviewees—Carmen was 18,

Heather was 21 and Gabriella, who was sexually assaulted as a child, was 29 the first time she had consensual sex—push the average age for first-time intercourse in this decade to a little older than 17.

For comparison, 20 was the average age for women in their thirties to begin having consensual sex, and in that decade the average was also affected by someone molested as a child. That woman—Tonya—waited until age 28 before choosing a partner.

For women in their fifties, 18½ was the average age for "the first time," while 60-somethings came in at 17½. Each decade, of course, contains late bloomers and early adopters.

HURRAH FOR HORNINESS!

Women in their forties—even the ones who lost their virginity at 14—mention desire and passion much more often than teens, twenties and 30-somethings, who instead cite curiosity and peer pressure when they recall their first time.

The 40-something ladies give good old-fashioned horniness its due.

"I had sex with my boyfriend, who was a year older, because I was always horny . . . always," says Linda, whose first time was at 14. "I thought it would feel good. I didn't think it was that big a deal, because my girlfriend who was 13 was doing it with her boyfriend [who was 24].[4] I wanted to see if it was as good as they talked about. It was curiosity too, sure. And it wasn't all that good. It was quick and not like I thought it was going to be. I thought it would be like having an orgasm by myself." (Linda,

---

4   Several women interviewed for *Kiss and Tell* describe having sex as minors with men somewhat or quite a bit older. Young women sometimes don't realize that adults who have sex with minors may face charges of criminal sexual conduct and statutory rape.

you may recall, began masturbating at 5 or 6.)

Even so, she doesn't rate the encounter a failure.

"I was being intimate with someone else; that turned me on enough to do it again, but it was not as satisfying as an orgasm. I didn't tell him, though. I didn't even tell him I was a virgin. Neither my brain nor my heart was right for any of that [having sex or a relationship]."

The couple stayed together for three months; then Linda found him sneaking around with other girls. She broke up feeling deeply betrayed and didn't have another partner for three years.

"Puppy love" is why Sassy said yes to having sex the first time. She and her boyfriend were both in ninth grade: "We weren't really dating; we were too young to date," she says, oblivious to the statement's irony.

She recalls that penetration hurt a little, but not for long.

"I was lubed up and ready; I was just *ready*."

Horny?

"Yes!" she enthuses.

The relationship was short-lived; Sassy met someone in tenth grade and he became her boyfriend—and sex partner—throughout high school.

Sage's first time—also at 14—was with her 15-year-old boyfriend.

"We were in my parents' bed," she recalls. (Sage's parents were separated and her mom worked days.) "I was young. I had the hormones and sensations. I was in love with him. I was sure I was going to have his babies someday," she says laughing.

"We would always go to the brink, which in Catholic terms was 'everything but.' On this particular day I did not blow the whistle. Yes, there was some Catholic guilt, but by the next day it was gone.

"We talked about it," she continues. "I loved him; he loved me. You can't put the cork in that bottle once it's opened."

The teens had a two-year relationship; Sage says he broke it off right before she turned 16. Her next lover was much older, in his twenties, "the epitome of a boy gone bad," and someone she dated on and off for five years.

Amy, another 40-something who had her first sexual relationship in ninth grade, says she had crushes on her female babysitters from the age of 6 or 7 and always knew she was gay.

"She was Filipino," Amy recalls fondly of her first. "We used to have sleepovers. You know that game where you write letters on your friend's back and they guess what you're writing? She'd be touching me and I'd think, 'How come I'm feeling the way I'm feeling?' Well, one thing led to another and the exploration began."

The two stayed together all through high school, but drifted apart when Amy left for college and her lover began to date guys.

Carmen was 18 and had been dating her future husband for five months when they first had sex. She carries happy memories of the occasion.

"I remember that day. We were at the beach, in the water, kissing . . . he was touching me. I was ready. We left the beach and went back to his place and had sex. For me it was anticipation, because I had never done it before. I knew I was in love with him. It was also a little disobedient. I'm from a Hispanic home, so I was pushing the envelope. I'd always listened to my parents; this was the first time I'd made a decision for myself and said, 'Hey, I'm going to do this.'"

Though the majority of interviewees recall that passion affected their decision to have sex that first time, a few did not succumb to a partner's advances because of overwhelming desire.

For Bonnie, who lost her virginity to a 19-year-old, "desire didn't play a part in it."

"I think it was more because I was 15 and any other girl my age already had. He was my boyfriend and it seemed like that was what I was supposed to do."

She thinks they'd been dating a few months when she said yes.

"It was mediocre," she recalls. We were at his apartment. It probably lasted 10 minutes."

Heather also denies feeling a passionate connection to her partner.

"I don't think I knew what horny was at that point," she notes.

Gabriella, who didn't unearth the memory of her father's early sexual molestation until adulthood, had sex consensually for the first time at age 29, on her honeymoon.

"When I got sex, I was thinking, 'That was it? This is sex? I don't really like it.'"

CASE STUDIES

Our interviews for the forties decade happen to encompass two women who starkly illustrate opposite ends of the desire spectrum—and to a certain extent, the guilt spectrum as well.

Gabriella, with only one consensual lover in her lifetime, wrestles to overcome the long-term effects of her controlling father's sexual abuse and sometimes wonders, "Can I redo my life?" A childhood anorexic, she still struggles with body image and low self-esteem.

Heather, who estimates 800 lifetime sexual partners, learned from being in a swingers' lifestyle in Los Angeles to "quit worrying about what other people think; we all have our flaws." The former call girl isn't burdened with guilt and doesn't second-guess her choices.

For their contrasting viewpoints, these women's stories are worth a closer look before we bid goodbye to the forties decade.

"A lot of women can't do what I do," Heather remarks. "I think like a man about sex, not like a woman. Meaning a lot of women will have sex and that makes them attached. If I want to have sex, I'll have sex. It doesn't matter about a relationship. I can not even know your name and say, 'Good-bye, I'm done.'"

Heather believes shyness initially held her back sexually: "Once you shed that, things are very different. Also, I realized I shouldn't have rules with myself about getting married or that you shouldn't have sex with too many people or you're a whore. I realized it really doesn't matter, and if you like something and it's not hurting anyone, who cares? It's *my* choice. And I'm not being fooled by someone who's pretending they like me so they can get in my pants."

Contrast that with Gabriella, who only now—eight years after her divorce—is opening to the idea of a second sexual partner.

"For the first time, I'm thinking I want to enjoy sex," she says, and seems surprised to hear herself speaking such words. "My friend says, 'Why do you deny the biggest pleasure in life to yourself?' I don't know. I don't have the answers. But you know what? I don't want to suffer again; I don't want to get hurt again."

She certainly has a multitude of hurts to overcome in this arena. For instance, her ex-husband piled insult on injury toward the end of their 13-year marriage by crudely requesting anal sex.

"He said that I was not tight anymore, so he wanted it tight again. I told him I'm not an object," she says with a tremulous laugh. "Now I'm laughing, but it made me cry for a long time. I tell him I have three kids; I cannot be as tight as the first time. I thought it was mean, disrespectful and nasty to say it."

Gabriella looks younger than her 48 years, with soft eyes, medium-length brown hair and a pretty figure. But since childhood, she's seen a different picture.

"I always feel ugly, like I'm not pretty enough. Only now, looking back, can I see I was cute. I don't want my daughter to follow in my path, to go through her whole life and wait till she's my age to realize she's cute now."

Though today Gabriella can see her childhood beauty, she's not able to recognize her 48-year-old appeal.

"Sometimes I think I want to know how it feels to have sex with someone else, even if it's not a permanent relationship. I'm not that ugly; I could maybe date. I have a friend from Cuba married to a man 10 years younger. She says if you have sex with only one person, it's like reading only one book in your life. She says I need to go out and find somebody. . . . She had fun when she was younger—and she doesn't regret it. I wish I could be that secure."

Given Gabriella's story, her low self-esteem is understandable.

Born in San Miguel, Mexico, she describes her young self as interested only in school, sitting on the front row of class and focusing exclusively on the teacher. Her first boyfriend was an admirer from high school who approached her when they began attending college together. After a year of carrying her books from class to the bus stop, he attempted to kiss her. It was only a peck, but Gabriella was horrified.

"I was 18, but it was like I was 10 years old," she says. "I told my girlfriend and she says, 'Are you crazy? Why are you freaking out?' I asked her if [the kiss] was okay, and she said of course."

A few days later she and her boyfriend shared a second, longer kiss.

"After that, he went to my father and asked if he could be my boyfriend. I was worried my father would be upset."

But the relationship was condoned, as long as the couple's dates were confined to Sunday afternoons between 1 and 4—just enough time for a movie and the bus ride home.

"I was taught I couldn't have sex with anybody until I got married. My culture said if I had sex with him, he would dump me and I would have nothing to hold him with."

After six years, the couple became engaged and was planning an autumn wedding—but in the spring it all fell apart.

Gabriella found pictures of her fiancé relaxing poolside with friends on a business trip and made a scene. "My idea was he could not have fun with anyone but me. I was very insecure.

"I regretted it the rest of my life because he was the love of my life," she mourns. "My insecurities pulled us apart."

Gabriella's father made things worse by telling her no other men would ever be allowed at the house, and by comparing her to a prostitute.

"I was 24," she recalls. "I knew I was too old already [for another chance]. By then, I'm supposed to be married with kids."

Gabriella moved to Canada for schooling, then Florida, where she eventually met her husband, a roofer four years her junior. They married when she was 29.

"Sex was always just, 'Do whatever you want to do,'" she explains. "I had to fake it because I wasn't enjoying it."

Her husband would tell her, "You just have sex with me because you think, 'The poor stupid man, he needs sex because he hasn't had it for a month.'"

Though Gabriella would deny it, she knew it was true.

Her moment of revelation, the event that brought her childhood trauma to light, occurred one day six years into her marriage, when her mother called from Mexico.

"My mom told me that she and my father were going to come to Florida, come stay with us, [since] we had residency. She said my father can work with my husband as a roofer and she can take care of the babies [Gabriella's children were toddlers], so I can work full-time. When she said that, I said, 'No, I don't want my father to come.' But I didn't tell her why. I was so scared he was going to do something to my kids."

Her long-suppressed memories were only half-formed, but a therapist has since told Gabriella that her fierce maternal instinct to protect her children was likely the only thing strong enough to strip the veil from her eyes about her father's abuse.

Soon after the call, when Gabriella's memories began surfacing, she consulted a priest to ask whether she should share her fears with her husband.

"The priest says maybe I misunderstood what my dad did. So I told my parents they could come, but I told my husband, 'I think my father molested me many years ago. Do not leave my kids alone with my father. Never.' He started laughing and said I was crazy. 'You are his favorite,' he said."

Gabriella was too unsure of her memories to contradict her husband, so her parents moved in. It was a miserable time, with her father smoking in the house in blatant defiance of Gabriella's request that he smoke outdoors in deference to her son's asthma. His machismo was offended by what he saw as a daughter's disrespect.

"It was a big mess," Gabriella reports, but the upshot was that she stood her ground about the smoking and her parents eventually went back to Mexico.

Only later, during therapy, did she unravel the tightly wound tendrils of delusion that she developed to protect herself from the horror of her father's abuse.

"Don't doubt that it happened," the therapist told her. "A person who has never experienced abuse doesn't suddenly say, 'I think this happened.' It probably happened many times, and you only remember the last time. The love for your kids was bigger than the block in your head keeping you from thinking about it. The cover you put over the abuse fell down so you could see the danger your father posed to your kids."

"*That's* why I didn't have a boyfriend, *that's* why I freaked out when he tried to kiss me and that's why I don't want to have sex," Gabriella finally realized. "Everything makes sense now."

But the ramifications of childhood rape may never truly end.

HealthyPlace.com, a mental health website run by an independent media company, lists the 10 most common sexual symptoms after sexual abuse or sexual assault as:

1. Avoiding or being afraid of sex
2. Approaching sex as an obligation
3. Experiencing negative feelings such as anger, disgust, or guilt with touch
4. Having difficulty becoming aroused or feeling sensation
5. Feeling emotionally distant or not present during sex
6. Experiencing intrusive or disturbing sexual thoughts and images
7. Engaging in compulsive or inappropriate sexual behaviors
8. Experiencing difficulty establishing or maintaining an intimate relationship
9. Experiencing vaginal pain or orgasmic difficulties
10. Experiencing erectile or ejaculatory difficulties

With almost one in five American women reporting an attempted or completed rape at some time in their lives (according to the 2011 National Intimate Partner and Sexual Violence Survey conducted by the Centers for Disease and Control Prevention) it's important to know that molested women may experience the return of body memories while engaging in sexual activity with another person.

Gabriella's general lack of desire is classic after abuse, even though her memories didn't resurface until her father's presence threatened her children.

After her divorce, Gabriella had a serious discussion with her sister about taking care of her children should something happen to Gabriella. Her sibling didn't question why Gabriella stipulated that their father not be given access to the children, which prompted Gabriella to tell her sister of the abuse.

"She is like, 'Okay.' And she is quiet," relates Gabriella. "She believed me. And then she tells me he tried with her. She was 16 . . . he was drunk. He pushed her down on the bed, but she pushed him back . . . she was heavy then. I wonder," says Gabriella, choking on a sob, "why I *didn't*?"

Such questions are for therapists, and Gabriella reports that on this subject her therapist points out that her sister was 16, whereas Gabriella was 9, or likely younger.

Subsequent observations concerning her family history have led Gabriella to expand her opinion of her father's philandering.

"I think he started with his sisters," she says, referencing conversations in which her aunts have hinted at such abuse and asked Gabriella probing questions about her alienation from the family. "[They say] Dad was always with other women, including a cousin. I think my mom has to know. But it's so hurtful; she's not going to say anything."

Gabriella hasn't reached the point of deciding to confront her father.

"For what?" she asks. "I haven't seen him in eight years."

A glimmer of hope for Gabriella's future has recently surfaced. Though her children and job obligations restrict her opportunities to meet men, in the past year she's occasionally had a cup of coffee with a friend and coworker.

"Last time, when he was talking, I was looking at his mouth, and I was thinking it was a cute mouth," she confides. "He has a little bit of beard, and he talks so proper and nice. I catch myself focusing on his mouth. And then I'm like, 'No! What am I thinking?'"

Ask what situation she ideally envisions in five years and Gabriella's answer shows measured optimism.

"I'd like to have somebody to maybe have sex with . . . and also for chatting. But I don't see somebody living with me. I don't like that."

***

Though Heather and Gabriella share the experience of a conservative childhood, Heather experienced no abuse, and, early on, the two women's stories head in opposite directions.

Raised in Miami, Heather now says she's embarrassed to admit she's from South Florida. She's moved back after two decades in California, but clearly still considers the West Coast her true home.

"I'm from L.A.," she says with pride. "The mentality there is different. It's very open. I used to go to swinger parties, so that may be the difference. When you're in the lifestyle, you're very open."

It was in Los Angeles that Heather realized, "Being shy isn't

a plus, and by being open, you learn from others' experiences
and that changes your life drastically."

She doesn't recall exactly how she got started in the lifestyle.
"I got an idea in my head one day and went online. I found
a party and went."

She paints a picture of uninhibited, nonjudgmental scenes,
where people danced in various states of undress and where
intimate touching by both strangers and friends was common-
place. She attended both house parties and clubs, and recalls
L.A. Couples as a favorite haunt.

"People would take their shirts off, they might grab each
other . . . and you could be totally yourself without worrying about anything. No one [at a straight party] would touch
your boobs or put his hand down your pants, but there it was
fine. You could be free to have a good time. They had themed
rooms—like an Aladdin room—and people might wander in
and have sex. If someone was watching we didn't care."

She insists it was a safe scene: "Everyone used condoms in
the clubs; they had bowls with condoms and lubes outside the
rooms. Nobody tried to have sex without condoms. If that happened, you'd tell the staff and they'd never be allowed back. It
was very controlled like that."

Heather notes that she scrupulously enforced safe sex at
clubs, and also when she worked as a prostitute. "Sometimes
I'd use two condoms; I always brought the condoms. I've never
once caught anything from working or the lifestyle. I've always
been careful."

She displays no evidence of feeling exploited during her
time in the lifestyle or as a call girl. Toward the end of her time
in L.A., she recalls dating three guys fairly regularly, plus others
she might hook up with.

"Before I left, I was with a different guy every night," she says nostalgically. "I should never have left. I realize now I just needed a vacation. I should not have moved."

Today, Heather lives with James, a man she met in 2005.

"It wasn't supposed to be anything more than casual sex," she explains. "I'm the type of person who likes to be with different partners. But he just kind of stayed, and the problem is, I'm still the same kind of person. For a while we were great, but the novelty wears off. We're still friendly and we do everything together. We live like a married couple, but now I really don't want to be with him. He's more of a hassle. I've suggested we stay in separate rooms, be roommates, and we can both date. But he doesn't want to do that."

So Heather has begun seeing another man on the side, which she's uncomfortable with, having never kept any of her sexual exploits secret from a partner.

Part of Heather's disenchantment with James stems from the low libido he contended with several years ago.

"His testosterone level went down and he lost his desire," she relates. "I told him, 'Either do something about it or I'm going elsewhere.' I waited for a couple of years; it hurt my feelings that he wouldn't get the treatment. He knows how sexually active I am, but he'd push me away. I knew it had nothing to do with me not being desirable; it was him not caring enough to take care of me. And that's mean. He made it like there was something wrong with me. It wasn't a concern to him."

Then about a year ago, Heather met Mario.

"For months I'd walk around thinking about him," she says. "He stimulated me so much; it's probably the most incredible sex I've ever had."

When it rains, it pours, so naturally James has recently opted to receive testosterone therapy and "is like a stud again," according to Heather.

Still, her fantasies focus on Mario, not James.

"This guy can kiss like no other," she enthuses. "He's really into foreplay and doesn't go right for the treasure. He knows how to please a woman, and he loves to give oral sex. I ask him how he knows what I want, and he says it's because he really enjoys it. James does [oral sex] because I like it, not because he likes it. Now [James] is all like, 'I can't do this; my nose gets stuffy; I can't breathe.'"

Heather, who says she's never liked watching porn ("it just looks gross to me"), has never been into masturbation and doesn't own a vibrator.

"Once I got sexually active," she explains, "I always had guys around. I never did that stuff."

There is no one position she favors during sex, but her quickest route to orgasm is finger stimulation during intercourse.

Like most women, she finds it hard to orgasm through intercourse—"It's happened to me a few times, but not a ton."

With Mario, she likes to be on top.

"It depends on the mood and how things are going—and it depends on who you're with," she says. "It's crazy with Mario; the orgasms are deep and different and multiple. It's so intense."

Heather notes that Mario is married and is also seeing one of her friends. The friend, who raves to Heather about what a great lover Mario is, doesn't realize he's seeing Heather as well.

Uninhibited Heather did have a monogamous L.A. boyfriend for two years, who she thought was "the one." It was before she entered the lifestyle, she says.

"Mark and I didn't have sex for several dates—because I didn't want to: we were *dating*. That's different than if I just want to go have a good time. I think maybe I'm strange, but if I want to have a relationship, that's different. I take it slowly. I want to get to know you first before I have sex."

Heather says she doesn't know just how she changed to be so different from the reticent girl she was in her early twenties. Asking what's had the most impact on her sexuality elicits this response: "I think maybe just being open to things and not worrying about what people think. Life is too short. We need to make every day worthwhile. I don't worry about repercussions or what anyone thinks."

Now if only she could share a bit of that powerful sense of self with Gabriella, we'd consider it a more just world.

DECADES OF DESIRE:
THE FIFTIES

SOME READERS MAY BE SURPRISED BY THE NUMBER OF WOMEN in their fifties who respond "right now" when asked, "When's the best sex of your life?"

But if you think about it, it makes sense. Why wouldn't the empty nests many women enjoy in this decade create both renewed desire and a receptive environment for sexual experimentation?

Of the 50-something women I interviewed in depth, 60 percent said they were enjoying their best sex now; the other 40 percent all named their twenties or thirties as their decades of greatest sexual delight.

That more women like the sex they're having in their fifties than the sex of their twenties goes against long-held notions about postmenopausal sex. So who are these women?

Elizabeth is single now and looks 10 years younger than her stated 58; she has sexy dark eyes, a great figure, luscious red hair and sparkly flip-flops. We talk on her screened-in porch about the sexual reawakening she experienced when her second child left the nest.

"From [age] 50 to now is when I've probably learned the

most about sex," she says. "I'm doing things I would never have done before. But I figured, 'How long are you going to wait to try that, to be open?' I realized sex is something you should never shun. You should enjoy it, because it's a wonderful feeling, and why wouldn't you want to have it?"

She once worried what other people would say if they knew of her sexual exploits, but Elizabeth has since decided it's no one else's business.

"It's your private world," she says. "I always worried you couldn't have sex on the first date. [She was a virgin until her honeymoon at age 22.] But I've learned you don't have to have rules; you can have any kind of sex you want without worrying."

Her contemporaries echo this frame of mind. Candy, who filled out the survey in her fifties but had turned 61 by the time of our interview, raised four children with her husband, Jim, a part-time associate pastor. She remembers a period of 15 to 20 years when she was consistently too tired for sex.

That's all changed.

"There's not the pressure of, 'The kids are in bed; we have five minutes!'" she offers. "Now we have more time for each other. I can stop cooking and we can just sit on the couch. I don't have four kids I have to cook for."

Bianca, 57 and recovering remarkably quickly from back surgery when we talked, praises the prowess of her second husband, but gives the highest marks to Miguel, her current 48-year-old lover.

"This guy has more positions than Carter has pills," she divulges. "He does everything to make sure he satisfies me and *then* himself. He says, 'How is that for you? Do you like this better or that better?' I never saw anything like it in my life. He cares more about me, which is unusual for a man."

Bianca even says it seems like she's having more sex than any other time in her life.

This isn't to say the fifties decade doesn't bring challenges. For example, Christina, a single, retired educator who's 55, hasn't had sex in more than two years, and reports that lately even her vibrator doesn't bring her to orgasm.

But the idea that women in this decade aren't interested in and actively pursuing satisfying sex lives is dead wrong.

A total of 289 women in their fifties participated in our survey, making it the second-largest decade represented in this book; only the forties, with 300 subjects, is larger.

Overall, the interviewees are fit, fashionable, independent and talkative. Most display a quality we like to refer to as "juicy," meaning their zest for life is strong and their interest in life's exciting possibilities hasn't waned.

THE POWER OF THE PILL

A marked difference emerges between fifties and sixties women in the realm of premarital pregnancy, which makes us wonder whether the juiciness referenced above might be related to a woman's ability to enjoy sex without the constant threat of pregnancy.

Not a single interviewee in her fifties got married as a pregnant teenager, while 33 percent of our 60-something interviewees did just that. Another 33 percent of the sixties spokeswomen became pregnant on their honeymoons, indicating that while birth control pills were attainable, in theory, to that older decade of women, in practice the pill's cultural and practical assimilation took years.

Fifty-something women were clearly more in charge of their fertility; the majority of women we spoke to used birth control pills for contraception for varying lengths of time.

Renee, for example, who's 52 and the mother of two grown children, took birth control pills all through college and up until she wanted children, which wasn't until age 29. Marie, a 55-year-old lesbian with no children, visited Planned Parenthood for a prescription at 16, when she started having sex. She was on the pill for a decade, throughout several affairs and a yearlong marriage when she was 25. (She was 35 when she first fell in love with a woman.)

Candy, the associate pastor's wife and eventual mom of four, began using the pill around age 16 to regulate her painful periods. She was an on-again, off-again user, but stayed on them during a yearlong first marriage, and resumed their use later when she met Jim.

"I didn't want children until I met him," she explains, indicating that reliable birth control enabled her to have children with the man she *chose*.

Just 10 percent of the sixties women are childless, but 30 percent of our 50-something interviewees opted not to have children, and it's reasonable to assume the pill facilitated those decisions. Choosing to remain childless were Christina, a bisexual woman who never married, and Alexa, a 55-year-old artist with a toned body and a flair for the dramatic.

"I never wanted children," Alexa says, sitting in her studio alongside the vibrant, colorful paintings she's known for. "My mom was mentally ill, no question about it, and I guess I was afraid that dysfunction would be passed on. I didn't want to jeopardize a child."

Though she used birth control from age 14 to 33, Alexa's efforts to avoid conception were unsuccessful.

"I got pregnant while on the pill," she shares. "My gynecologist called me Fertile Myrtle. I took them like clockwork, but you know how they say they're 99 percent effective? I was the 1 percent."

Alexa had three abortions and one miscarriage during her two marriages, one of which lasted two years, the other two decades.

"That's why I go crazy when they talk about reversing *Roe v. Wade*," she says.

Not everyone from this decade relied on the pill.

Rosemary, who married at 23 and lost her virginity on her honeymoon, trusted condoms. She and husband, John, who've now been married 39 years, were raised Catholic. They had their only child when Rosemary was 28.

"We were *very* careful," she emphasizes.

During her childbearing years, Elizabeth (she of the luscious red hair) also eschewed birth control pills, and Bianca, a mother of two, says she never took them because her mother was convinced the pill caused her breast cancer. Nevertheless, Bianca developed breast cancer in her mid-forties, and had a double mastectomy in 1999, between her two marriages.

While the pill certainly facilitated these women's ability to enjoy sex with less worry of pregnancy, a related factor was also at play in this decade.

The in-depth interviews revealed that women now in their fifties were the first to fully inhabit the expanding sexual freedoms available to their gender due to the sexual revolution. This decade serves as the dividing line: In general, women 60 and older come across as somewhat more conflicted about their sexual development, and occasionally a bit removed from it.

But the 50-somethings have embraced the new sexual world order; many of them divorced the husbands who disappointed them and sought satisfaction elsewhere. They came of age at a time when premarital sex no longer carried the stigma it once had and when experimentation was more widespread. Not surprisingly, fewer women in this decade were virgins when they married. The country's shifting cultural standards meant that taking multiple partners didn't disgrace a woman—and our interviewees took their cues accordingly.

FIRST-TIME TALES

When asked for their famous "deflowering" stories, women of all ages say sex wasn't what they were expecting. Only a few women I spoke with looked back on their first time with a look of dreamy sentimentality. Nerves and a woman's physiology, coupled with a too-eager young partner, don't generally produce fireworks.

For this decade, 18½ is the average age of when our interviewees first had sex. Several waited till their early twenties, including Nina, a 59-year-old widow.

Nina married at 25, but lost her virginity to her future husband two years earlier. Raised in Turkey, where girls' virtues are fiercely guarded, she says her sexual daring was very unusual in her culture.

"That's because I had a foreign boyfriend," she explains. "He was 17 years older than me, a big, blue-eyed German Hungarian, really handsome, a big American executive. He selected me to teach him the language. Before you know it, I was so in love with him. He was so charming."

However, there was no question of Nina visiting businessman Lee at his hotel: "The doormen would call the police," she says. "Girls have to stay a virgin."

Lee eventually visited Nina in Italy when she was a student, and continued his wooing.

"I did not desire sex," Nina confesses. "I did not know about it. I liked the romantic part, the kissing, the flowers, to love and be loved. He was very patient. He had to have sex every day, so in between he was a playboy.

"I told him, 'How could you do that?' And he said, 'I love you, but I'm a guy and I have my needs.' It wasn't a very good explanation, but it was logical."

A bit of theatrics ensued before Nina was willing to have sex with Lee. When he balked at marrying her because of a messy divorce in his past, Nina became engaged to a young man who worshiped her.

"That's when I realized you have to love the person. Before [meeting] Lee, I figured you grew up, got married and had kids. . . . I never even thought about falling in love. But I realized, 'My God, I can't even kiss [my fiancé].' I realized I loved Lee."

So Nina created a huge scandal by canceling her engagement, and then went to Germany to continue her education.

"That's when Lee came back. He found out I'd broken the engagement. He bought all these flowers and came to the university to see me.

"And *that's* when I lost it!" she says of her virginity.

In contrast to Nina and others, Bianca and Alexa each tried out sex at 15.

Alexa had an adventurous encounter with an older guy, maybe 19 or 20, when traveling in Germany with her parents.

"He was a big, strong swimmer, and (we met) on a rustic island with lots of sticks and leaves and bugs on the ground."

They solved the prickly ground cover problem by having upright sex, and Alexa says no pain was involved, and no orgasm.

"So after the sex, we swam back around to the other side of the island. . . . 'Hi, Mom. Hi, Dad,'" she says, grinning.

Bianca, who began dating at 13, gave in to her future husband after two years together: "I knew I was going to marry him, even at 15."

She didn't have an orgasm and wasn't impressed.

"I bled," she recalls. "I didn't know what the heck was going on. I remember thinking, 'What's all the hype about?' I must have been nervous."

Candy, although older, was another disappointed first-timer. "I was 19 and in college in Florida. He was a Greek guy . . . a liar! He was engaged and didn't tell me about it."

They dated for a couple of months before she said yes.

"It was more from pressure than desire; there was no climax," she recalls. "I met my future husband on the rebound, and I remember the first time I had sex with him thinking, 'Wow, this is what it's supposed to be like.'"

Katrina, a tall, beautifully sculpted mother of two who first had sex at age 17, was likewise underwhelmed.

"It was a one-night stand, basically; I cheated myself out of it; I gave it away."

Elizabeth, who waited till her wedding night for intercourse, had dated her husband for five years and done "everything but."

Despite having orgasms during oral sex from age 17 on, she doesn't remember being initially turned on by intercourse (at 22).

"It was short . . . it was loving," she says. "I remember being scared a little, like it would hurt. It didn't really, but I also didn't think, 'Oh, that was great; let's try it again!'"

Elizabeth now covets the responsiveness of her 17-year-old body: "All he had to do sometimes was touch my breasts and

I'd come. I wish I could have that body back! I wish [my body] lasted and could take all that stimulation now."

Rosemary, another of those who waited, has better memories of her honeymoon than Elizabeth.

"It was hard to get his penis in my vagina," she recalls. "It hurt, but I did climax; I remember that."

Rosemary, who sports silver jewelry and exudes an earth mother demeanor, began masturbating around age 10, and says she had lots of orgasms before she married, but had no idea what they were.

The first time she had an orgasm with John, they were making out in the car and his elbow was touching her vaginal area.

"Those were the hot-sex days, when we'd steam up the car. I was so turned on. And I told him to stop, but he said, 'Oh, come on, it's okay.' And we did. And I had an orgasm."

A casually placed (or perhaps strategic?) elbow isn't the route to orgasm men often envision for their partners, but women have specific routes that lead them to climax, and it's usually not penetration.

LET'S (NOT) HEAR IT FOR PENETRATION

Women like intercourse; no doubt about it. But when they talk about what brings them to climax, it doesn't top many lists.

In fact, of this decade's 289 survey respondents, just six women answered "deep penetration" when asked for their quickest route to orgasm. One more answered "slow penetration."

Clitoral stimulation (of no specified type) was the number one answer, garnering 27 percent of the total. Oral sex was the quickest route for 23 percent of 50-something women, while 17.5 percent answered masturbation or manual clitoral stimulation. Another 12 percent of fifties women specified a vibrator as their quickest route to orgasm.

Of the sampling of 50-something women we interviewed in depth, oral sex was mentioned most frequently, followed by masturbation or a combination of stimuli, such as breasts and clitoris simultaneously.

Marie likes oral sex, then penetration with a sex toy, and Rosemary is thrilled with the vibrator her husband gave her when his libido waned due to antianxiety medication.

"It was the best gift he ever gave me," Rosemary shares. "I have given one (the Brookstone Pressure Point vibrator) to so many people. It's so small and packs into my toiletry bag. I call it a girl's best friend.

"We shouldn't have to struggle," she says of her demographic. "As you get older, it's harder [to climax] because those nerve endings die off in your nipples and your vagina. They aren't as easily stimulated as when you're younger. With the vibrator, it's like instantaneous, sometimes too fast!"

(Dr. Whelihan confirms Rosemary's conclusion: "Nerve endings can indeed get a bit dull with aging, so the more intense stimulation of a vibrator provides a faster 'wake up!'")

Rosemary, who taught sex education to high school students for 10 years, praises her husband for branching out to find a fresh approach to their sexual playtime.

"He was so uninhibited about using it during intercourse, and finding a position where we could use it and have intercourse at the same time," she says. These days, the couple has intercourse about once a month, but plays with the vibrator together every week or so.

DIMINISHED DRIVE

Never-married Christina has also turned to a vibrator lately, but is frustrated by her low libido and inability to reach orgasm.

"It worries me because I would like to have a relationship," she says, "and men want sex even at 80 . . . but I seem to have lost my sex drive somewhere along the line. It went from really good to really bad really fast."

Christina was about 50 the last time she had a sexual relationship during which she had orgasms; she believes her troubles originated with the early onset of perimenopause, which occurred at age 35.

"Although I was able to have good orgasms till about 40 or 41, the frequency dropped drastically after that," she says. "I attribute that to the hormones decreasing. I did hormone therapy, including birth control pills and natural hormones. Then I hit menopause at age 52, which took a while to get through."

She no longer even expects orgasms.

"It's not like when you were young and the desire was always there. I had a high sex drive. Guys love a woman who loves sex, and I was always that woman. I've had to adjust my identity . . . it's been a major loss."

Christina, who guesses she's slept with 8 or 9 men in her life and 5 women, has worked diligently to retain her libido.

"I've been trying for the last couple of years to keep it stimulated by masturbating, because I've heard that's a good technique to keep things going. But in the last year or so I cannot have an orgasm at all, no matter what I do, and that is very discouraging. It's like you're touching yourself but there's nothing. You're just doing it to be doing it. Not that I give up easily either. I try. But now, I admit, I don't expect to have an orgasm, so I don't try."

Elizabeth uses computer-dating sites to create a very active social life, but she too complains of similar issues.

"Sometimes I can't even have orgasms with myself. I use a

vibrator more often than my fingers; it's quicker. But then other times, I'll just be thinking about sex with a guy, and I can just touch myself and it's like I'm a virgin; it feels like the first time. I'll come within a minute. Then sometimes it's never."

Elizabeth does climax regularly with her current partner of 6 months. And her husband of 22 years total (she married him twice) "knew how to give me an orgasm . . . there was never had trouble with that."

But no woman likes to realize the equipment isn't as sharp as it once was.

"Menopause absolutely takes the desire away," asserts Marie, 55, who has been with her female partner for seven years. "The hot flashes dry you up down there. I have to use a lubricant all the time now. But my personal opinion: A lot more foreplay would help that situation."

Marie, who estimates she's been with 25 guys and four females, says she and her partner have sex every couple of months, and that she could go without for a year and not have it bother her.

"It started to die down at 48, because menopause—I call it mental-pause—took my drive away. I've had the patch; I've had this and I've had that. I don't want any more drugs. I will still smoke a little weed now and then, but I will *not* put anything else in my body," says Marie, who was in prison for 4½ years in the nineties on drug charges.

Marie also bemoans what she calls mind-wandering during sex.

"That's why people watch dirty movies during sex, I'm telling you. It's to keep their minds from wandering."

She notes that her weight is an issue as well.

"Being overweight takes the drive away," she shares. "When

you get overweight, you get tired and you get embarrassed. You don't want to take your clothes off . . . you get shy."

While menopause certainly lessens desire in some women, for others the change of life brings an uptick. Renee, Nina and Alexa all reported heightened libidos in their late forties and fifties.

MORE, PLEASE

Renee, a pretty dark-haired woman now separated from her husband of 26 years, said she experienced a sexual reawakening around age 48 or 49.

"It was caused by hormones," she says. "I told my husband I wanted more sex. . . . That's when he bought me a vibrator, which never got opened!" (She didn't care for a substitute.)

Looking back, Renee can see that her change of life had no effect on her husband or his dedication to work.

"He owns his own business and works seven days a week," she says. In addition, he's overweight and has some health issues.

"His sex drive just wasn't the same as mine."

During the past decade, the couple's relationship became increasingly platonic, and when their kids left the nest, Renee's lust led her to begin the first of three extramarital affairs.

"It's like the desire to have sex was coming out of my pores," she says. "It wasn't to the point of addiction, but it was strong. Maybe having sex outside my marriage enhanced those feelings of desire. I definitely feel it's eased off now, at 52, and is not at the level it was."

Renee is still having periods, but classifies herself as premenopausal. Instead of her previous rate of intercourse with her husband every six or seven months, she and her current lover have sex several times whenever they get together, at least weekly.

Nina, who was widowed at age 47, is another late-life bloomer, saying she learned the most about her libido in the years following her husband's death.

"I wasn't a stockbroker anymore; I became a real estate agent and started wearing more casual clothes . . . nice dresses, maybe sleeveless, more bare, you know? I would notice people looking at me. . . . I got all this attention. So I think maybe I'm pretty. What did I know? I was a content married woman and hadn't noticed before. I began discovering my sexuality in my late 40s, for goodness' sakes."

Nina's reawakening came from the discovery that she could take control of her sex life. As a much younger, foreign wife, she slid into the trophy-wife role without thinking—dressing the part, playing hostess at their parties and always welcoming her husband's sexual advances.

"I did sex because I knew it's what he wants, but it's not *my* sex, do you see? It was just a gift. . . . He called me an iceberg sometimes. I loved him, but [after a while] it wasn't a sex love anymore. It was loyalty, commitment, whatever."

Though now in a four-year relationship, Nina says she's had about 20 lovers since her husband passed away.

"I had to like them," she says. "I won't pick up a stranger. I had to respect them. And they have to be yummy-looking. It doesn't matter if I'm not yummy; *they* have to be yummy. If I decided it wouldn't work out, I would break up. I had these raging hormones; I'm glad I didn't have that hormone rage when I was younger."

Nina believes, in her case, that hormones allow her to sustain her healthy libido.

"When I wasn't getting good hormone therapy [during menopause], it was painful," she reports. "I couldn't get wet.

[Sex] was like taking a dry stick and putting it inside of your body. That's a big reason why I stopped dating people."

Today that's changed.

"I'm having very good hormone therapy now," says Nina, who's been taking bioidenticals for the past two years. "I feel happier and sexier than I did 10 years ago. I take a gel in my cheek twice a day . . . it slowly absorbs."

Nina says it eliminated all her symptoms, including hot flashes, and improved her bone density.

"But it gets me very horny." She laughs. "The doctor says that's a good thing, but my boyfriend thinks I'm a sex maniac."

Elizabeth is another 50-something woman who sings the praises of estrogen and progesterone, because, "I don't want to ever give up sexual desire. Life is too boring to give that up too."

Dr. Mo says without estrogen and testosterone (the hormones that are excitatory for sex), post-menopausal women may well feel empty and barren as a desert.

"In many cases, hormones can make women feel youthful and alive," she says, "and each patient should discuss this with her gynecologist."

Though Alexa, the artist, isn't taking hormones, she is another in this decade who reports a midlife improvement in her already healthy libido.

"My sexual desire has increased and become more satisfying," she says. "As I age and become more relaxed with who I am, the sexual experience is more desirable than it's ever been."

ADVENTUROUS ALEXA

Alexa has short, spiky hair, an athlete's body and an artist's bon vivant attitude. She considers herself bisexual and enjoyed 16 years of the swinger lifestyle with Greg, her second husband.

Her libido has stayed reliably high throughout her life, except for a period when Greg was terminally ill.

She readily acknowledges her strong sex drive, occasionally referring to herself as "a real pig," which she cheerfully translates as someone greedy for sex.

"Sometimes I think there's something wrong with me," says Alexa, who takes no hormones but suspects her testosterone level is higher than average. "I asked Dr. Whelihan if I'm abnormal because of the size of my clitoris. It's like I'm a woman in a man's body. I know I have a large clitoris from all the men: They're like, 'What *is* this?'"

Alexa's clitoris is about as big as a thumb when aroused; she notes that her current partner, a bisexual man, loves it and swears he's never seen one like it.

"Dr. Whelihan made me feel better by saying it's normal but rare," Alexa shares. "I feel more accepting now. She said to just enjoy myself."

There is no normal size for the clitoris, notes Dr. Whelihan, and it is subject to both genetic variation and external modifiers. External influences include things such as adrenal gland malfunction, but also perhaps the practice of applying testosterone directly to the clitoris. That's usually not recommended, because sometimes the effects are irreversible, she warns.

Genetic variations include race, notes the doctor, and in study groups comprised of women with large clitorises, African-American women are found in greater numbers.

"The majority of women have a two-centimeter clitoral 'button' length," she says. "The diameter is about two to four millimeters, but what's more important than size is the understanding that the clitoris has 'legs,' or crura, which extend down around the sides of the vagina under the labia. These 'legs' cause the labia's puffiness when aroused."

In Alexa's case, the doctor says she may have more active—or free —testosterone than other women, which could make her good at sports and might have caused her sex drive to develop at an earlier age than some.

Alexa was a self-described jock growing up in Michigan: She swam, played volleyball and ice-skated. As described earlier, she lost her virginity in Germany at 15, and had several other sexual partners in high school. She married at 24, and divorced 22 months later. At 31 she married Greg (who was 12 years her senior), and they stayed together until he died in 2008.

"We worked together, vacationed together, even started to look alike," she relates. "We wore the same clothes, cut our hair the same . . . people thought we were brother and sister. We were both Capricorns; we wanted to resolve issues so they wouldn't come around again."

She learned the most about sex during their marriage, she says.

NOT AN EXCLUSIVE MARRIAGE

After they'd been together seven years, Alexa and Greg decided to swing. (Only one other interviewee—Heather, from the forties chapter—told us she was part of the swinger lifestyle.)

"We did swinging with other couples, *not* wife swapping," clarifies Alexa. "In other words, our rule was to swing with the other couple in the room at the same time. We were not going out with other people and dating separately."

Alexa and Greg switched partners or had group sex with multiple couples, almost always at swing club resorts.

"You can go to destinations in, say, the Caribbean or Costa Rica where there are other people of that desire," she explains, noting that four- and five-star hotels offer all-inclusive packages. "It'd be some fuck party for a week; we'd spend five or ten grand. And they have vendors there where you can buy cool clothes for the swing clubs. There would be a leather night, for instance .. . the women dress like little sluts and whores."

As for the sex itself, Alexa says, "Girls would have sex with each other . . . sometimes the men would have oral sex with each other, but not anal sex, because typically we were with other heterosexual couples. That's what I experienced."

Alexa adds that most of the people on such vacations are very attractive by anyone's standards.

"It's a turn-on to see your mate having sex with someone else, and swinging couples feel the same way. Then you go back and have sex with your partner and it's exciting all over again."

The knowledge she gained from the swinger lifestyle remains.

"I learned that people are sexual beings and that hetero-sexual relationships with a single partner are probably a very unrealistic option for a human being in our society, because we *are* sexual beings. I believe it's okay to want something on the side that will end up stimulating the relationship with the person you're most intimate with on a daily basis."

Today, four years into her widowhood, Alexa's sex life centers around a bisexual man she referenced in her survey under "the best sex of your life." They are approaching three years together, although Tony still lives with his long-term male partner.

"We call it friends with benefits. We have sex—usually once a day, maybe twice—whenever he's in town. Every now and then we try for three, but that's only happened a couple of times. It's hard to do for a man who's going to be 65 soon."

Tony lives nearby and is Alexa's personal trainer; occasionally they even travel together. Ask her for the one thing she wishes he wouldn't do, and Alexa draws a blank.

"He can do whatever he wants. There's nothing I don't like. He's a dream come true."

And then . . . "I take that back. He won't kiss my lips because I smoke cigarettes. That's my punishment; he cannot stand cigarettes. It's in my skin, so he says, 'No way, no way.' But my pussy, no problem!

"I do wish he would kiss me, but if I quit smoking, that'll be my reward. If I get to kiss him, then I'll really fall in love."

Alexa, who quit drinking last year, says Tony was instrumental in her sobriety. When Greg was terminally ill, her drinking increased, and when he died, Alexa says she became a "stay-at-home drunk."

"When I moved to Florida [and took up with Tony], he would never have sex with me when I was shit-faced. That helped me to quit. I didn't want to lose respect from him as a friend . . . and I don't want to hurt the people I love."

Since alcohol is the factor Alexa cites as affecting her sex drive the most, she's still adjusting to the changes its absence brings.

"Alcohol lowered my inhibitions and increased my desire. I'm a pretty open person. . . . I don't have a lot of inhibitions, and alcohol lowered whatever inhibitions were left. And because of that euphoric feeling, my body was able to relax even more and be more stimulated sexually. I had higher, more intense levels of orgasms, including actual ejaculation."

Alexa took this information to Dr. Whelihan as well, who again informed her that female ejaculation is rare, but not abnormal.

"It's gross," Alexa disclaims. "It's a mess . . . all these liquids." But the sensation is worth it. Alexa explains that—for her—

previous orgasms during a lovemaking session make ejaculation more likely.

"The orgasms get more and more intense. If there's oral sex first or intercourse that brings me to orgasm, then [the ejaculation] is icing on the cake. That's when I'm a real pig. It hasn't happened since I stopped drinking. . . . I haven't tried, though."

Because she spent 16 years as a swinger, with house parties hosting 10 to 15 couples, Alexa's lifetime number may be the highest we found—as many as 1,000. (Heather, interviewed in the forties chapter, estimated a total of 800, largely due to her years as a high-priced call girl.)

"It's over a hundred but less than a thousand." Alexa laughs.

Could she narrow it down?

"Well, I hit a hundred my first year in college, so I didn't count after that. It's probably several hundred. . . . I hope it's not over a thousand! Isn't that disgusting? But the human body is such a beautiful creation."

Perhaps we'll just declare Heather and Alexa tied and leave it at that.

The remainder of the 50-something interviewees averaged 13 lovers in their lifetime, from one (Rosemary) to 29 (Marie).

A FEW MORE NUMBERS

Equally revealing as these lifetime numbers are the figures about how frequently women have sex—which dramatically changes depending on the partner.

Bianca says she had sex with her first husband (of 20 years) once a month; with her second husband (of four years) twice a week; and with her current lover (of seven years) five times a week.

"With my first husband, if you're lucky and he's in a good

mood, it was once a month," she says. "But if he blamed me for something or was mad, well, one time we went two years. He withheld sex as a punishment because he knew I liked having sex with him and knew it would piss me off if he didn't.

"He was so routine, it was like you're in the army: first this way, then this. My second husband was better. But I've never met anyone like Miguel. I always thought that you had to please them. I never could have imagined that someone would care enough to see that you get satisfied."

It takes work to keep passion alive in long-term marriages, and not surprisingly, Bianca wasn't the only woman to express dissatisfaction regarding sex with former husbands.

"The first time I was married to my husband, we had sex three or four times a week," Elizabeth says. "It was always a chore. He wanted sex before we went out for the evening, so he didn't have to be horny all night. I'd be like, 'Don't people go out and have a nice evening and come back and have sex after?' I felt like he was raping me for seven years."

When Elizabeth divorced Kevin, she had several lovers, including a man she says taught her more about sex than anyone else.

"There was curiosity there; I was not a virgin anymore."

After five years of single life, Elizabeth remarried the father of her children.

"It was a good marriage that time; it was definitely more loving," she says. "We were kinder; we spoke softly to each other."

The sex was better too.

"We were more compatible since I'd been out there on my own; I could look at it positively."

Her second marriage to Kevin lasted 15 years, roughly twice as long as the first; she's now been single for eight years, and dates frequently using online services Match.com and JDate.

These days, she and her current lover have sex every time they're together, perhaps three times a week, she says.

Marie—who's been with her partner for seven years and has sex infrequently now—was married for a year at age 25 to Joey, a man she'd lived with since she was 19. They started out having sex three to four times a week, but dropped to a couple of times a week.

They divorced when she caught him cheating, but both were using cocaine then, which likely affected their sex life.

Marie recalls having zero orgasms with Joey—she labels him "the minuteman"—and though she didn't masturbate as a child and "couldn't care less about it," she occasionally resorted to it during that time.

Marie's bitterness was compounded when she contracted chlamydia from Joey, presumably from his extramarital activities.

After their divorce, Marie dated other men, not taking a female lover until she was 35. She wasn't consciously looking for a woman, and says she didn't care about Andi's gender when she met her through work.

"What attracted me was her eyes," she reminisces. "She was seven or eight years younger and kind of looked like a guy. After we had sex, that did it. It restoked my fire. I'd been doing drugs and was depressed.

"We had sex every day, three times a day . . . and I was having an orgasm every time. That's why I kept going back for more."

Marie says during this time period she learned how to have an orgasm with a partner.

"Guys never did it for me, because they just wanted to get off and that was it. Kissing wasn't even an option with a guy."

The pair moved in together, but after just six months, Marie was arrested on drug charges.

"We were torn apart," Marie says. "But I think the reason I was attracted to her was maybe God was getting me primed for a new lifestyle."

In prison, Marie met a new lover, and they served most of their sentences in the same institution, then stayed in touch when they were assigned to different facilities. When Marie was released, she set up house, and when her girlfriend was released a couple of years later, they resumed their sexual relationship, and lived together another three years.

"She was cheating on me with a guy," Marie relates. "I told her it was going to happen and it did. She used me as a scapegoat and tore me up."

When that relationship ended, Marie was celibate for about five years.

"I also didn't drink or do drugs of any kind, even pot. . . . I was scared to," she says.

She says she used the time to become more comfortable with herself. She went out dancing, had fun, went to gay bars hoping to meet someone, but never did.

"You can't really make love to another person if you don't love yourself," she says. "And I learned to love who I was. I don't care if you're tall or short or fat or you smoke or whatever, you'd better love yourself."

Bringing this full circle, to the question of how frequently our interviewees have sex, Marie reveals that she and her partner (whom she describes as a kind, caring, loving person) now make love every couple of months. Because of her previously mentioned libido drop, which arrived with menopause, Marie says now she "could go a year and it wouldn't bother me at all."

LOVE, LUST AND LONGEVITY

So what can sustain desire as decades pass in the life of a woman? Younger women don't approach this subject with the same intensity the fifties women do.

Nina and Elizabeth have already made the case for hormones: Both insist that their supplements enable them to keep the sexual fires burning. But it's worth noting that for almost all women, what *creates* desire and what *sustains* it are vastly different.

Alexa, for instance, says she's turned on by a man's physical fitness, his ability to make eye contact, his voice and "his dick."

Ask her what sustains desire, and the answer is "intellectual compatibility.

"The mind is an interesting sex organ," she elaborates. "The brain is the largest sex organ, and a long-term relationship encompasses intellectual compatibility, trust and respect of your partner. *That's* a turn-on. You grow to trust their opinion because they're smart . . . there's a mutual-admiration-society aspect. I think that's what keeps a relationship going.

"The brain—how someone thinks—that won't wear off. Whereas if someone's pretty and has a good body, but when they open their mouth stupid things come out . . . ugh, they're a turnoff."

Elizabeth's desire is stimulated by seeing others kissing, by her lover's body and smell, and by thinking about how wonderful it feels to have him inside her. She says "thinking about how good it feels" is also part of sustaining desire, but there's more.

"It's communication," she emphasizes. "You need to be able to talk about what you like and be comfortable expressing yourself and your desires. I also have to feel wanted, definitely. And, for me, a relationship is not sustainable unless it is monogamous. If you don't feel like you're special, desire can't be sustained. I *have* to feel that."

She adds that a strong sex drive "can be the glue that holds you together, but you need to have the foundation of the relationship. . . . Having a good relationship is what drives me to the bedroom."

Renee, the woman separated from her husband, mentions communication as well. Though she lists foreplay, wine and music as things that stimulate her, it's a different combination that sustains desire.

"A connection emotionally with the person," she insists. "If somebody cares about you, and works at keeping things exciting, you're more apt to sustain desire. . . . . It doesn't become old or stagnant. You have to communicate and work at keeping it fresh. It starts in the mind."

Bianca also notes discrepancies between what causes initial attraction and the requirements for sustaining a long-term relationship.

She writes that "anything" stimulates her desire with Miguel, and specifically cites his "gentle, soft-spoken ways . . . when he looks at me with those puppy eyes."

But as she thinks back over her marriages, she can see that her seven-year affair with Miguel is built on much more.

"I think it's the attitude, the friendship that you have," she muses. "My first husband, the communication was the worst. He never wanted to do anything with me and the kids, so I could have cared less about having sex with him. My second husband, we used to do everything together, even food shopping. We'd laugh while going up and down the aisles like idiots. We loved the same movies . . . we had fun. So my desire for him didn't change from the day I met him to the day we got divorced.

"With Miguel, we talk about anything and everything. I help him a lot because he speaks broken English. I'm always there to help him. . . . I do his [accounting] books for him. He sees me as a genuine friend. He sees how much I go out of my way for him and don't ask for anything in return. I think he gets overwhelmed by that. I don't think he's ever had a genuine friend."

Christina, one of our interviewees who experiences low desire, says visual stimuli (porn) can turn her on, though she rarely watches now.

"I need clitoral stimulation in order to orgasm, but lately even that's not doing it. . . . I need breast or anal stimulation."

As for what sustains desire? "Just being in love with them," she answers. "Wanting to please them."

Rosemary cites "thoughts of sex and positions" and "my husband's body and penis" as her turn-ons, but, like Christina, love is her pick for what sustains desire.

"I think it's loving someone, and the physical attraction . . . knowing that it's going to be satisfying."

Marie and Candy (whose husband is the associate pastor) are the only interviewees whose answers indicate that creating and sustaining desire feel the same to them.

Marie's survey lists dancing and smoking pot as stimulants; her answer to what sustains desire merely expands on those same stimuli.

"Vacations, special moments or events . . . but mostly dancing, drinking, smoking pot. That's the only thing that keeps me going, and we don't do much of that these days. But I'm not gonna run out the door anymore [and fool around]. I have a guy friend I hang out with and do stuff with—everything except sex. I still like to have fun. It's still embedded in me to go out dancing, talk to people. Music is what moves me . . . arouses me."

Candy's answers to both questions are also similar; both are rooted in gratitude. To "What stimulates your desire?" she responds, "Thinking about how blessed I am . . . the wonderful man I married. He is the most flattering husband, and he does it genuinely. As far as stimulating sexually, it's stopping and thinking about it and getting in the mood . . . just sitting on the couch, touching, caressing, making the time for each other. Too often, people don't stop and make the time. I heard somewhere that women are Crock-Pots and men are microwaves, and I think that's true. We have to warm up and think our way into it before we can get into it. Men just have to visualize and open their eyes and they're in the mood."

As to what sustains desire, Candy says it's "appreciating the man that I've got and seeing how blessed I am. I don't use the word *luck*. God has blessed our relationship over the years to show you *can* stick together, you *can* make it through."

She then notes that early in their marriage, Jim had a one-night stand, which he confessed to Candy much later, when their four children were young.

"Even then, as rough as it was, we made it through. [The indiscretion] was before we had a personal relationship with Jesus Christ. We call it BC, Before Christ. We've had hard times; we even went through personal bankruptcy a while back. But we didn't point fingers. God is the glue that's held us together. It's a three-way covenant."

WOMEN NEED A FOCUS

For single women in their fifties, unfamiliar challenges arise as they contemplate new relationships.

"I don't want 'just sex' anymore," says Christina, who considered her libido very strong until she was 41. "It's sad but true.

Now I would require an attraction or emotional attachment to the person before sex, which is very hard as we all get older, because none of us look the way we did—men or women. I still see myself as a younger person, but I look in the mirror and say, 'Who is that? My mother's here.'"

The women in this age group don't generally experience free-floating desire, that need to have sex just to satisfy biological urgings. While men this age (with normal testosterone levels) may still be in the market for casual sex, the women are less so. And as Christina mentions, the initial attractors (broad shoulders, thick hair, strong arms) that draw women to men and fan the flames of desire are less apparent in aging males.

Another factor for a woman starting over is her ability to relax sufficiently to reach orgasm. Without the assurance of a climax—and often without much estrogen—Rosemary asserts, "Nothing is *driving* women in their fifties to look for sex!"

To her friends who tell her they never climax, she says, "If you aren't having orgasms, why would you even want to do it?"

But then she shares what's clearly an oft-told story to prove that fairy-tale endings can be found.

"I know a couple from my church . . . they've been married two years now. She was a widow and hadn't had sex in 15 years; he was a widower. They fell in love and married and they have a very strong sexual relationship. The first year they were married they were very active, and she told me she couldn't believe how her body was responding to sex again. She said, 'Oh, my gosh! I can't believe how wet I am!'"

Rosemary laughs and insists this woman has more sex than she does. "And she's 74 years old! Isn't that wonderful? So I guess it can happen. That flow can come back."

Since Rosemary was the only 50-something interviewee

with a single lover, her story of how her own sexual desire has evolved holds interest.

"Sex wasn't that great when I was younger," she confesses, "probably because I was inexperienced [though her husband was not a virgin]. I'd never had sex before, so it was a learning process for me . . . getting to learn my body and not being inhibited with my husband. I'm totally uninhibited with him now. We discovered I had a dry vagina and we had to learn how to make it better lubricated. It was a learning process to discover what to use, what not to use, what kind of condoms."

The couple also experimented to find positions that were enjoyable for both, and they watched porn as well.

"That was always a turn-on," she shares. "We started doing that in our late twenties and we still do it occasionally, because he needs the stimulation." As previously noted, her husband, John, takes a mood-leveler medication for depression and anxiety that negatively affects his libido.

"We try to work around [his lack of sex drive]; sometimes we'll watch X-rated movies and that helps him to get stimulated. The times when he can't get an erection at all, we get out the vibrator and he'll satisfy me that way. It's funny how the vibrator works for girls but not for guys. He doesn't enjoy it at all."

This phase of her sex life isn't Rosemary's favorite, but she has faith things will turn around.

"It's definitely a change and it sucks. I miss the closeness of sex, but hopefully we'll get back there. I tell him, 'I like you to rub me, touch me, make physical contact. We don't have to have sex all the time but I still want closeness.' We have that little chat all the time. I have to keep reminding him."

Despite the couple's current challenges, Rosemary's success rate for sexual satisfaction is high. She says in the early days of her marriage, she achieved orgasms about 95 percent of the time; today's it's 100 percent. "And it's easier now, because of the toys."

SO, HOW 'BOUT THOSE ORGASMS?

Christina's inability to orgasm notwithstanding, many of our interviewees report frequently satisfying encounters. Elizabeth says she has climaxes all the time, and Bianca estimates 90 percent of the time. (She achieved orgasms with her first husband about 25 percent of the time, and with her second husband all the time.

Alexa had orgasms about half the time with her first husband and then 99 percent of the time with her second husband. Katrina says she climaxes whenever her husband performs oral sex, which she estimates is about 80 percent of the times they make love.

Marie denies ever achieving orgasm with her husband, but says that with her first female lover, she climaxed every time.

Candy's success rate was 25 percent with husband number one, and is now 50 percent with Jim.

"It's so much more relaxed," she says, though she notes that she's sometimes wondering whether his Viagra pill is going to work.

"As my husband has gotten older and it's more of a challenge [for him] to keep an erection, playing lollipop [oral sex] is a way to help him keep his erection. Oral sex is more about foreplay than for orgasms for both of us.

"If he doesn't have a climax it's okay for him. I will have one or two; then the next time, I'm not so focused on having a climax, and I'll just enjoy pleasing him." Jim does still have orgasms, she says, about half the time.

Candy says she tried AndroGel a couple of years ago to increase her testosterone, but didn't see the desired rise in her libido.

"I still don't have the desire I wish I did, but it's sure fun to play around. He has the desire; he always comes up behind me in the kitchen—we conceived one of our children on the kitchen counter! As you get older, to me, it's exciting to still have a husband who desires me."

Being desired is mentioned as an aphrodisiac by women of all ages, and a look at how Katrina's doubts about her husband's fidelity affect her interest in sex demonstrates that the opposing principle is also true.

THERE'S ANOTHER WOMAN

Marie, as mentioned before, left her husband when she caught him cheating. Nina didn't find out her husband had fooled around until after his death, so she was at least spared the pain of deciding whether to stay or end the relationship.

That difficult choice is exactly the one now faced by Katrina.

When she met Norm, Katrina was 34 and living with her dad, trying to get back on her feet and recovering from a disappointing five-month relationship with a married man. Her distrust of men is compounded by her first marriage—if you can even call it that.

Though they wed at a courthouse in a ceremony she had every reason to believe was legal, Katrina was shortly approached by an attorney who said her new husband was already married.

"He was a sociopath and a liar. He took all my money. It was not even a legal marriage. He committed bigamy and there's no record of it."

Their split led to Katrina's move to Florida, and the aforementioned disillusionment. Three months after that breakup, she met Norm, who was three years younger and had been married twice.

Katrina was going to school and working nights when she met Norm. His generous ways won her over, but after just two weeks of dating, Norm saw the realities of her schedule and told her it wasn't going to work because she had no time for him.

"He came up with the idea of me quitting and working for him around the house, with him paying all the bills so we could see each other every day. I told him I wasn't ready to have sex. . . . I'd already had sex with a couple of guys since I moved down here. But he said he was willing to wait till I was ready."

So she quit the job, began cleaning his house, doing laundry, writing his checks and cooking meals. About a month later, they had sex: "He took me to a hotel on the ocean and made it real special. We spent the weekend up there."

Back then, Katrina says, "I loved having sex with him. He's a sexual dog; he needs lots of sex . . . I was accommodating."

After they tied the knot, Katrina discovered she'd married a man just like her stepdad, who put his job first. She takes care of the couple's son and daughter; for him there is lots of travel and overtime . . . and there are the women. For years, she chafed over Norm's close relationship with his secretary, and now she's feeling threatened by Mary, another work acquaintance.

"It happened before with his secretary." She sighs. "He says there's no sex. But both women divorced their husbands over him; they say their husbands are beating them up. The last one even came to my house. I give them my clothes; I've taken care of their kids."

While she tries to be supportive, Katrina has become increasingly conflicted as to why Norm brings women into their circle this way. Though she's been vocal about her disapproval of their relationship, she recently blew up when she found out Norm paid to take Mary along on an out-of-state business trip.

Though he insists Mary is a friend, he's put a lock on his phone and keeps his computer with him at all times.

"Plus he deletes all his e-mails," Katrina says. "I told him, 'I can't trust you.' All I've known is men who cheat on their wives. I question everything."

When she confronts Norm, he answers with, "I'm not fucking her. I want you."

It's not enough, and Katrina doesn't desire him the way she once did. She often uses alcohol as a prelude to sex.

She wonders now what attracted her to Norm.

"He's not romantic . . . and he can be selfish. I don't know if I stay with him for the kids . . . the obligation. He does provide a very good living for us. The kids go to private school. I see all those attributes in him."

She doesn't want to believe the worst.

"He always rolls over and rubs my feet after sex, every time. And I think, 'A man like this *couldn't* be having an affair with Mary.' But I still feel I can't trust him. . . . I will put off kissing him or hugging him. So I guess I'm withholding because of that."

UNEXPECTED BISEXUAL VIEWPOINTS

In each decade, as candidates were selected for my in-depth interviews, Dr. Mo and I strove to select lesbian women, wanting their voices included. In most age groups, we were able to find lesbians to go on the record about their desire.

Marie is the lesbian voice we expected to explore in this chapter; however, two additional women in their fifties—who had given no indication on their surveys of being gay—told me they were bisexual during their interviews.

Their stories were very different but equally fascinating: Christina dated women exclusively during her twenties, but has since returned to a heterosexual lifestyle; Alexa began having sex with women only after she and her husband entered the swinger lifestyle when she was in her late thirties.

Christina lost her virginity to her first boyfriend, Joe, at age 16 and dated him for 4½ years. She met him at 15 and did heavy petting for a year.

"I had sex because I was madly in love with him," she says. "There's no doubt that I was horny, but a big part of it was that I was crazy about him. It wasn't that I felt he was going to leave me if I didn't have sex with him."

Their first time was in the back seat of his car, and Christina didn't climax. She had many orgasms with him during oral sex, she says, just not with intercourse.

Christina says she's been diagnosed with dyspareunia and has a small vagina, so "a large penis isn't a good thing for me."

Dyspareunia—pain with intercourse—can be either insertional pain or deep pain, according to Dr. Whelihan.

"The causes for each are different, so it's important to investigate and treat accordingly," she explains. "In this age group, insertional pain is more prevalent; it's most often attributed to estrogen deficiency, which causes the tissue to become thinner, nonelastic and more likely to tear."

The doctor says this is easily remedied with a small amount of estradiol on the skin of the vaginal opening two times a week.

"Of note," adds the doc mischievously, "for those ladies who prefer no medication, having three orgasms a week or more will maintain the youthfulness of the vulva and vagina—so get to work!"

Does Christina think her dyspareunia influenced her attraction to women?

"Not a lot, but I do think maybe a little . . . maybe it was subconscious. I guess there's a part of me that wondered why I was having so much trouble. I later found out Joe was huge. I thought everybody looked like that. [She estimates his penis was eight or nine inches long.] That was tough, especially as your first. It's not just the length, but the girth."

Christina broke up with Joe after their freshman year of college, though for years she thought they would marry.

"We had named all our kids, the whole nine yards," she says. "Fortunately we started arguing—he was the jealous type—and didn't follow through with marriage."

Christina had another male lover as well, but then began a lesbian relationship in college and dated women exclusively for a decade.

Her first lover was a couple of years older.

"I think it became a relationship only due to alcohol," she says. "I had felt feelings of attraction to women and fantasized about it, but I wouldn't have had the nerve to act on them. She made the first move. . . . It was her first lesbian experience as well. We had been drinking. I don't think I would have been able to get involved in a lesbian relationship without that. Emotionally we got along really well. I liked her a lot.

"In my twenties and into my early thirties, I considered myself bisexual," she says, "but in the past decade, when I think about making love to another woman, I find it unappealing. So I would not consider myself to be bisexual anymore. However, when I was younger, I was open to not only sex with either gender, but a relationship."

At age 30, Christina started dating a man.

"It wasn't a gender issue," she clarifies. "It was a relationship issue. I happened to be attracted to him as a person. At that time in my life, the circumstances were right. I didn't just wake up one day and say, 'I'm going to go back to men.'"

After that relationship, Christina dated one more woman, and that was the last time. She says she stopped being interested in women around age 31.

"I think women have much more in common with other women," she says. "I have a hard time understanding men; I truly do. I understand women much better, but there's not that physical attraction any longer. There's still an emotional attraction, but not a physical one."

Alexa, on the other hand, is attracted to women physically, but has had no exclusive, long-term relationship with one. She considers herself bisexual, having engaged in multiple encounters with women in groups through the years, sometimes with one other couple, sometimes with several other couples.

Though she's now a widow, during the years when she and her husband, Greg, were swingers, Alexa says she looked forward to sex with the women: "Women know women's bodies a lot better than most men, I would say."

However, she never had sex without Greg's presence.

"He loved to watch two women getting it on," she recalls. "For guys, it's like their favorite fantasy."

IS THREE A CROWD?

Threesomes are indeed a fantasy for many men, but do women embrace it with the same enthusiasm? Since bisexuality shows up unexpectedly for 50-somethings, I also asked about threesomes.

Neither Renee nor Rosemary had participated in one, while

Marie's survey told us the best sex of her life was during a three-some—with two men.

"It's the only threesome I ever did," she says. "We all met when partying. It was the excitement of having them both and not being able to choose which one of them I wanted."

She laughs at the idea that a lesbian's best sex was with men.

"I guess I'm a lesbian. You know that joke . . . 'What do they call a late-life lesbian? A slow learner!'"

Nina has never had a threesome or a lesbian experience, perhaps because oral sex isn't her favorite thing.

"Oral sex is not something that has to be done to stimulate me. There are women who like that, and some men just start right away with oral sex, but it's just part of everything; it's not a necessity to me. It's sweet; it's nice, of course . . . a nice, hot tongue. But I've never had an orgasm just by oral sex."

She says her lack of interest in women or threesomes may stem from her conservative upbringing.

"I've been approached many times by lesbian women. I like a dick and I like a guy. One said, 'There are ways a woman can satisfy a woman that a man can't.' I said, 'I doubt it.' To me, no way a woman could turn me on. I am respectful of their sexuality, but it's not mine."

Bianca says she and Miguel once had a threesome with another woman.

"But I didn't touch her and she didn't touch me; we just touched him. I probably won't do it again. First of all, I hate my body; I have so many scars [from the double mastectomy], and I don't want to be in the company of a woman who has a beautiful bust, you know what I mean? I always keep my shirt on when we fool around, and [Miguel] respects that. He doesn't tell me to take it off. He knows why I don't want to remove it.

"One day I did show him this side," she says, pointing to her right breast. "It doesn't faze him. That's another thing I love about him."

ANAL, ANYONE?

Although a moderate number of 50-something women named anal sex as the one thing they wish their partner would not attempt, other responses (such as "being insensitive to my needs" or "rushing to intercourse") scored nearly as high. With so many women overall singling out the practice of anal sex as undesirable, I frequently asked for opinions about it during the in-depth interviews.

The majority of fifties women I queried have no interest in anal sex. However, some indicated they enjoy variations of anal stimulation, and others said they're willing to do it occasionally for their partner. More rarely, women told us they find anal sex very arousing in certain situations.

Renee says she tried it with her husband once or twice and isn't a fan; she hasn't allowed any other lover to try. Rosemary says she and her husband never tried anal sex, that she doesn't have a desire for it, "but apparently he doesn't either."

Bianca says anal sex is the one thing she won't let Miguel do: "He's tried, but he's too big for me. I didn't have anal sex with my husbands either."

Candy says in their early years she and Jim played with anal sex, "but it wasn't that pleasurable or that arousing. Neither of us had a climax that way. And it was uncomfortable, so it's like, why even go that way?"

Nina cannot think about anal sex without wincing. "I'm not curious and no one is asking me. In many countries in Asia and the Middle East where girls have to be virgins, I know some would do anal sex [instead]. No women really like anal sex, do they? I think men who like it aren't necessarily homosexual; they just want a tight place. But it's not hygienic. It's not the cleanest place of the body."

Elizabeth doesn't have anal sex often. "I only did it with one guy. I was crazy infatuated with him. It was good, but I don't think I'd want to do it on a regular basis. If I'm not lubricated I'm not going to enjoy it. Then it's, 'Get your fingers out of me; that's annoying me.' I can't believe we're talking about this," she adds, grinning.

Alexa had a traumatic introduction to anal sex—her first husband raped her anally, causing her to leave him shortly after.

"I told him no, but he said, 'You're my wife; you're gonna do what I tell you to do.' I said, 'You married the wrong broad; we are all done.'

"He jammed me with no lube or anything—I cried and hid in the closet."

Nevertheless, she tried it later with other partners, and her opinion today is that if it feels good, do it.

"It can be enjoyable if it's done right, but I have to be extremely aroused and have had several vaginal orgasms before I can start stuffing something anally. And I have to be totally relaxed and trust my partner; otherwise I'll tense up, remembering thirty years ago. Your asshole has a myriad of sensitive nerve endings that are phenomenal. If you're really stimulated it's the ultimate. I'm all for it with proper preparation.

"But it's not sexy if it's not clean," she continues. "You've got to do the enema. I'm funny about how things smell; I like my partner well groomed and clean; that's what turns me on."

Christina considers anal stimulation as one of the things she learned she enjoyed during her twenties, when she embraced a lesbian lifestyle.

"I dated a guy once who explained to me it was an erogenous zone, and so I didn't feel so self-conscious about liking it," she says. "He only used his finger."

Her sole experience with anal penetration occurred when Christina was in her early forties: "I was drinking with a guy one time and we had too much; he ended up raping me anally, actually. We were having a relationship, and though I didn't break up with him over it, we didn't date for long after. I guess I gave him the benefit of the doubt because we were both so drunk."

Katrina says her husband, Norm, wants anal sex, but she's rarely willing to oblige.

"He'll joke about it, but I've got to be really, really drunk. . . . Maybe twice a year, I'm willing. I'll get a Brazilian wax to please him, but maybe it's the stigma. I just don't want anal sex. My mom, who's very open about sex, told me she'd never do that and to be careful of it."

KEEPING IT ALIVE

So women in their fifties have experience with both rejuvenated sex lives and those that have grown cold. But by this age, most have gained an understanding of and reached a level of contentment about their sexuality.

"We have to work on our relationships constantly or they become stale," says Candy, who chooses commitment despite the challenges. "[Long-term marriages] aren't fresh. The fresh role is so much more appealing."

Those women who leave a failed relationship often find their libidos reborn. The natural surge of dopamine that a new lover can create is one of the primary reasons women stray.

"Sex with my husband got old and stale," says Renee, who's

separated now. "When you have someone you're in love with and you're not consumed by responsibilities, you can express a desire that perhaps has been pent-up."

Whether it's a woman like Nina, who rediscovered passion as a widow, or one like Rosemary, who is lovingly dealing with her husband's decreased libido, 50-somethings are deliberately choosing the paths to desire they wish to travel.

This decade is surely a time of transition, as women deal with work stress, empty nests and the challenges of menopause. But our interview subjects demonstrate openness, willingness and the most dramatic understanding so far of their own sexuality—as well as an eagerness to express it with their partners. Nothing in their candid revelations speaks to inhibition. They talk of children, death and divorce, yes, but when given the forum, they also express an abiding love of sex.

While the general consensus of society is that the older you get, the worse your sex life becomes, this notion needs updating. In her role as a sexual expert, Dr. Whelihan says men constantly tell her that women in their fifties "don't want to do it."

She uses one of her favorite lines: "Perhaps it's not that women have low desire; they may just have low desire for the sex they are having."

Based on the adventurous stories shared by this decade's representatives, it seems society might do well to reflect on its own biases about sex before assuming all is lost for women this age.

DECADES OF DESIRE:
THE SIXTIES

THE TERM "SIXTIES" HOLDS DUAL MEANING FOR WOMEN IN THIS decade: It both describes their age and identifies the "peace and love" decade that played such a monumental role in their individual histories.

Today's 60-something women were graduating from high school in the 1960s, a decade in which winds of change were sweeping the country, promising no less than an idyllic Age of Aquarius. The notion of a Prince Charming coming to rescue every girl lost favor, but only sketchy new scenarios arose to replace the debunked fairy tales. Teenage girls who had sex were still labeled slutty, and though talk of "the pill" was rampant, few high schoolers could get their hands on it. But even they understood "free love" to be code for "more sex."

Every teenage girl of the time was attuned to—and absorbing—the overt cues of the era, along with their powerful subliminal messages. It was a heady time.

Our survey gathers statistics from 193 women in this pivotal decade. The in-depth interviewees fall into three general categories: those who remain married to their first love and only sexual partner; those who took new partners after widowhood;

and those who divorced and subsequently experienced periods of sexual renaissance or experimentation. (Only Kay, 69, a happily married lesbian who had sex with men earlier in her life, doesn't fit neatly into any of these categories.)

Directly or indirectly, all the women interviewed in-depth for this chapter talk about the effect of the sixties on their sex lives. Just 20 percent remain married to their first husbands, a statistic that points to the obvious transition society was making in its acceptance of divorce and the likelihood of multiple sexual partners.

A clear dividing line can be seen in sexual activity between women in their sixties and seventies: Just one interviewee in the seventies decade had more than 10 partners, while 50 percent of our sixties women topped that number—and 30 percent had more than 30 lovers. Only Jana, 68, who lost her virginity on her wedding night, and Dianne, 64, who's struggling with loss of desire, remain married to their sole sexual partner.

Interestingly, no sixties interviewee disclosed having an extramarital affair. And almost all moved straight from their parents' house into a home with their husband, after either high school or college.

Our sixties ladies began sexual activity at 17½ on average, as compared to 18½ for our seventies interviewees. While Kay, at 14, had a pleasurable first encounter with a 16-year-old girl that led to orgasm, several others recall their loss of virginity as somewhat traumatic.

Trudy, a vivacious 66-year-old with short blond hair, stylish glasses and a cute, compact figure, doesn't carry fond memories of going all the way.

"That first time threw me into a state of incredible guilt, even though I'd been doing all the heavy petting," she says. "I couldn't even get up and go to school the next day. My mother finally took me to a psychologist, but I didn't tell her either. I was afraid she'd tell my mother."

Trudy's mom had drilled into her daughter that sex was only for married people. But after dating her boyfriend for six months, she gave in one day after school on the floor of her parents' house.

"That was the end of it. I guess I just couldn't say no anymore. I was crazy about the guy. But actually, intercourse itself at that moment was sort of anticlimactic. I had done heavy petting with a former boyfriend [including mutual masturbation leading to orgasm], so I was like 'Where's my orgasm?'"

Still, Trudy recalls "horrendous guilt" afterward, which went on for several months. "I didn't want to disappoint my mother, though I was still having sex with him. Over the years, though, I worked it all out. I realized it was a crazy, old-fashioned idea."

Kylie, who's just married her third husband, was 19 and in nursing school the first time she had sex. Her partner was her high school sweetheart.

"We went parking," recalls the 63-year-old newlywed. "I probably said yes because I'd heard friends in the dorm talk about having sex with their boyfriends. My mom wouldn't discuss sex with me, so I had no concept of sex.

"But I really loved this man. Each time I was with him, it became more difficult to say no. I was so caught up in sexual attraction and passion. It's a different kind of passion when you're younger . . . raging hormones. I had been dying to have sex with him for a couple of years, but I'd been stopping myself.

"I didn't know what to expect. The first time was not great for me because it only lasted a short time. And he pulled out."

Nevertheless, Kylie got pregnant.

"We didn't know anything about timing," she says.

If our interviews are any indication, Kylie's receptive fertility is common for this age group, and illustrates that although birth control pills were available, their use was anything but widespread, and their adoption into general use was far from immediate.

As foreshadowed in the previous chapter, sixties women (again, based on our interviews) became pregnant out of wedlock most frequently, probably because reliable birth control had not yet catch up with the country's changing moral climate.

While no fifties spokeswomen got married while pregnant, 66 percent of our sixties interviewees became pregnant before marriage or on their honeymoon—although one woman miscarried. (Tighter moral strictures against premarital sex were applied when our seventies ladies were young; even so, 33 percent of those women married due to a pregnancy.)

"In 1966, when I graduated from high school, people didn't have sex," says Kylie. "A few girls in high school did, but they were bad girls. We labeled them as slutty. It just was not normal in those days to do that. Or maybe people weren't admitting to it. A couple of girls got pregnant in high school and everyone talked about it. My mother put such a fear of God into me that I wouldn't have considered coming home pregnant . . . although I did just that at 19. I remember that scene, with our parents deciding our future. We sat on the sofa like kindergarteners, holding hands and listening as they told us what we were going to do. He agreed to marry me . . . but once I had a miscarriage, that was that. My dad got transferred to Florida and he came to visit twice, but then it fizzled out."

Jackie, a pretty leasing manager for a commercial real estate development company, also became pregnant before marriage.

She had sex for the first time at age 17, as a senior in high school. "It was in a car, and it was nighttime," she remembers. "He had been pressuring me. I think I just caved. I'd had been dating him for two months. I think I thought—and he may have even said—that he was going to break up with me if I didn't. He had been with other girls. I do remember, in the car, he was sitting up and I was sitting on top of him facing him."

A few months later, Jackie says she had her first orgasm. And a few months after that, she became pregnant and they married.

MORE FIRSTS, MORE FERTILITY

Dianne, who's been married to her high school sweetheart for more than 45 years, also lost her virginity at 17, just prior to graduation. She became pregnant a few months later, over her college winter break, and married her boyfriend on Memorial Day weekend—four months pregnant.

"Back then the only birth control was condoms," she says. "The joke was that all the guys carried them in their wallets, but mine didn't. We'd been dating about a year.

"That first time we'd been at a farewell party for a friend of mine who was going to Vietnam. The end of the party was very somber. We went up the phone path—they kept it mowed in the woods—and dumped our blankets by the lake. One thing led to another, and that was that. I don't know if I was his first. Everybody wanted him. He was football, track, an actor; he was just a prize and an all-around nice guy."

Both kids were raised Catholic in upstate New York.

"We knew each other so well that [sex] was the natural next step," Dianne recalls. "But it happened a little sooner than we'd planned. We knew what we were doing; we weren't totally naive. We could have stopped, but we didn't want to. We felt like we loved each other and had talked about getting married after college."

Laura, 68, is a statuesque blonde who grew up in a small town in central Florida. She was carefully watched by her mom, and had sex the first time at 16, shortly before an early graduation from high school. In her crowd, 16 was not unusual for first-time sex, she reports. After dating a guy from a neighboring town for six months, she was ready.

"That night, I wanted him to be my boyfriend," Laura says. "I had dated a lot of different people I grew up with, but Rod was from out of town, and I wanted an out-of-town boyfriend. I was trying to force him to commit to me."

A difficult relationship with her mother led Laura to leave home as soon as possible; she entered college in another city at 17. She married Rod at age 20, and essentially got pregnant on her honeymoon, noting that they had used condoms up to that point. They divorced seven years and one son later.

"I didn't really enjoy sex that much when I was first having it," she says. "I didn't enjoy it for myself till I was into my thirties. It takes a while to get over all the taboos you're taught. Plus I had a crazy jealous husband who demanded sex. I lost sexual interest in him pretty quickly after we married because of the way he treated me—and cheated on me."

Leigh, who's 68 and originally from New Jersey, put off intercourse until her wedding night. She was 19; five months later she was pregnant.

"It happened pretty darn quick," she says. "To tell you the truth, I didn't know what happened. I was a baby myself. There was absolutely no talk of sex in my household. I never saw my parents holding hands or anything like that. My mother was extremely warm and loving, but my father was very standoffish and showed no emotion. Like all my generation, we learned about sex from school and talking."

Leigh and her husband, who died of a heart attack at age 35, had "done everything but" intercourse before they married.

"I was very young and naive when I got married," she relates. "I knew from nothing. He gave me books [about sex] to read, and the more I read the more I wanted to try and the happier he was with me . . . and the more books he'd buy!"

Though Leigh first held the impression that certain sexual acts were dirty, she eventually tried many new techniques in her marital bed.

"I assumed everyone did what I did. But when I became single and went into the dating world and started talking with girlfriends, I found I had so much more sexual intimacy with my husband than I realized."

For example, Leigh thought everyone had oral sex, but as a young widow at 31, she found none of her friends had tried it.

"They were broadening their experience [and considering it], but I'd had it in my marriage and thought everyone was doing it," she says. "I attribute that to my husband and the books. He just wanted me to learn that it is okay."

Jana, a small and lean 68-year-old with strong Catholic roots, waited until marriage for sex—and got pregnant at 22 on her honeymoon.

"I knew how to kiss and that kind of stuff," she says, "but there was no way we were going to have sex."

Jana's mother died when Jana was 16, and her father followed three years later. She had three younger brothers and struggled to assume the heavy responsibility of being head of a household.

"It was a big five years," she says of the time between her

mother's death and her marriage. "When Mike [her husband] came to us it was wonderful. He took a lot of the load," she says. Jana didn't experiment sexually with boys her age.

"My whole dating life was trying to find the right guy God meant for me to be with. I was looking for Prince Charming all through college and after. It wasn't about exploring sex; it was about finding the right guy."

And when she did date, she strove for honesty, mindful of her straightforward relationships with her brothers.

"You don't date somebody for the purpose of just having someone to go out with. You don't string them along; you tell them if you don't have a connection when you're dating. If you empathize with males you don't do that. It's not honest."

Jana identifies strongly with boys, because she wanted to be one throughout her childhood.

"If you were a boy you could do anything," she recalls, citing a time when strictures on proper activities for girls were only just beginning to loosen. "You could run and play and have freedom, which I did with my brothers. When you want to be a boy till your breasts start developing, you look at boys differently."

Tiny Jana says she lost 10 pounds during the stressful weeks leading up to her marriage. She talked with one girl at school about sex, but had very little information.

What with the wedding plans, a reception at her house, the bakery orders, taking the dogs to the vet and mopping the floors the night before the wedding, Jana says she just didn't think about sex until she and Mike stopped at a Fort Lauderdale restaurant on the way to Miami Beach for their honeymoon.

"I was going down the stairs to the ladies' room and it dawned on me what was going to happen: 'I'm not going to be a virgin anymore.' It hit me like a brick: 'I'm finally going to know what this is about.' I was not scared or happy. Just . . . 'It's with someone I love and this is it. Oh, wow.' I wanted to get married and Mike was the one, but I hadn't thought this far ahead.

"I had no desire on my wedding night," she says, noting that her first orgasm occurred almost a year later. "I only was going to do what we were supposed to do; I knew I wanted to be a good wife. I loved him, but there was not the desire for sex."

Sophia, a short, round woman with light brown hair who's just turned 70, remembers that Johnny Mathis was on the radio the first time she had sex.

"'Wild Is the Wind.' That song helped me make up my mind pretty fast." She laughs. "We were in my living room, because my parents were away visiting my sister in New Jersey. Opportunity was part of it. But it was nothing like what I expected lovemaking to be."

Barely 18, Sophia had been dating her boyfriend for three years. She's Jewish, and didn't realize how Catholicism affected his sexuality until he began frequenting confession whenever they were intimate.

What surprised her about lovemaking?

"It was the time span," she says, echoing disappointed women everywhere. "From the time you first kissed to the sexual act was too short."

Still, generous Sophia says that once guys learn not to rush, the lesson takes hold. At least that's been her experience with the three lovers of her life: the aforementioned boyfriend, her late husband (of 38 years) and a boyfriend of four years.

SAMPLING THE FREE LOVE OF THE '60s, AT THE PRICE OF A FAILED MARRIAGE

These first-time stories make it easy to see why the pill was poised to revolutionize the female sexual experience. Almost all the women I talked with were intensely fearful of premarital pregnancy, and several had those fears realized. Others became pregnant almost the second they married or shortly after.

"The '60s and free love was just beginning when I was a high school senior and in college," notes Kylie, "so the effects of that era weren't universally accepted by our age group. I think the majority of women my age didn't have the opportunity to date or have sexual experiences before we married. When I was a girl, my mother said she'd send the sheriff out looking for me if I was late—and she meant it."

Kylie's first marriage, at 21, lasted seven years; her second, at 31, lasted 18 years. But at 49, she finally got to relish sexual freedom.

"After my second marriage, it was my time to go out and have fun and have sex with different men. When I was younger I didn't get to experiment, and so this was my time for experimentation. I didn't have to answer to anyone. I didn't have obligations. My daughter was raised; I could do what I wanted. I even got my nipples pierced. A friend thought I was hypersexual, out of control. But I didn't think so."

Two other women—Laura and Jackie—also experienced a sexual renaissance of sorts once their marriages ended. Although the 1960s are revered as the sexual revolution decade, these women's stories prove that the era's loosened moral strictures took much longer to achieve widespread acceptance. Several interviewees only adopted a relaxed attitude concerning sex after their supposedly happily-ever-after marriages failed.

Laura, who estimates she's been with at least 50 or 60 lovers, had only had sex with her husband, Rod, when their marriage failed. She didn't cheat on her ex, but says she began dating the moment he moved out.

"It was 1969 or 1970 when we split. . . . I was out in California, working in the pharmaceutical industry. I had my share of one-night stands. It was the thing to do. There was no stigma attached to it—so I did. It was pretty much that way until AIDS.

"I learned the most [about sex] in my thirties and forties, during that San Francisco time period," Laura continues. "Then, by my forties, I had more committed relationships, serial monogamy. I learned more about relationships in general and how sex figured into that. It took me that long to get over my anger and resentment toward men in general. My husband was an alcoholic who raped and tormented me. I don't think I could see past all that until I was more mature."

Jackie, who was pregnant when she married her first lover at 18, had four children before the couple divorced. She married again at 39, to a man 15 years her junior. They stayed together 8½ years, and she says most of her 30 lovers have been since their divorce in 1992.

Though she had an active sex life with each husband, it wasn't until she was on her own that she learned the most about the nature of her sexuality.

"That's when I figured out what works best for me. I think it all had to do with not being so concerned with what they thought and more about what I want or what I need."

For Jackie, being free of the "relationship" aspect of marriage allowed her to concentrate on her sexual desires and how they were evolving.

"The more attracted I am to somebody, the more desire I have," she explains. "And the things that attract me to somebody have changed. When I was much younger, it's how cute they were. Now intelligence is a huge turn-on, and how a man treats me. Plus how good they are in bed, because if they're not good in bed, I don't want to have anything to do with them. I don't want to do any more teaching."

She recalls too much instruction being required with a couple of former boyfriends.

"To some degree you have to let them all know what you like, and the older I am, the less inhibited I've gotten about telling them, or showing them. But if they don't get it, forget it. One guy [whom she felt obliged to teach], I would show him how to kiss and he'd get it and he'd say, 'Wow,' and then he'd go right back to his old ways the next time I saw him."

Kylie expressed similar exasperation: After three dates with a divorcé of seven years, she asked why he would pull back after kissing her and begin talking about his ex-wife. He confessed to nervousness because it had been so long since he'd had sex. That was their last date.

"I don't want to be with a guy I have to teach how to have sex," she says. "There are other guys out there."

ONE MAN, ONE MARRIAGE

Among the 60-something women interviewed in-depth, Jana and Dianne remain married to their first partners. Jana, you'll recall, waited until her wedding night to have sex, while Dianne married Randy when she was four months pregnant. Both women were raised in the Catholic Church, as were their husbands. Jana has three sons; Dianne two daughters. But while Jana's sex life is improving slightly with age, health issues have robbed Dianne of her once-healthy libido, and she struggles to maintain intimacy with her beloved husband of 45 years.

The couple rarely has sex anymore; during our interview, Dianne reveals it's been seven months. At the dining room table of their comfortable home she compulsively folds and refolds a place mat, recounting the health crises she's battled. Her husband, Randy, the boy everyone wanted in high school, works outdoors in the vast yard to give us privacy.

Though pregnancy rushed them into marriage, theirs has proved to be a deep and lasting relationship, one in which she's stood by Randy during his treatment for testicular cancer and he's stood by her through multiple health crises that began with a life-changing accident. In 1973, Dianne's car was hit by a tractor-trailer pulling logs. The couple's 4-year-old daughter, their youngest, was almost killed, and two other children in her care suffered devastating injuries as well. Dianne's head was crushed, her jaw was broken in several places, one eye was crushed, her nose was broken and she suffered serious brain swelling. She couldn't drive for months, her hands didn't work and her jaw injuries caused speech difficulties. She choked often and couldn't chew.

A few months later, Randy was laid off, but fortunately found a new job.

And then, because "we handle each other a lot," Dianne explains, she found a knot on one of Randy's testicles. "It felt like a hard pea. That was 1974. He had his testicle removed and went through radiation." He recovered completely and soon moved into a good job as a plant engineer.

Meanwhile, Dianne's symptoms were multiplying, and the doctors said it was all in her head. She visited the oral surgeon who'd been putting her jaw and mouth back together.

"My eyes are falling down, I can't talk, my speech is off . . . and my oral surgeon says, 'What's happened to you?' It turns out I had myasthenia gravis, an autoimmune system disorder."

More patience and rehabilitation followed, for both Dianne

and her daughter, who recovered fully.

So when Randy's job gave them a chance to move to Texas in 1978, the couple took it, eager for a change of scenery.

"We were ready for some sunshine; we got a breath of fresh air," Dianne recalls. "That was our decade of delight."

Dianne writes on her survey that her best sex was with Randy in their early thirties, "during a period of frequent, hours-long foreplay and stop and start and finish together." She repeatedly uses the label *decade of delight*, a charming and appealing description.

"We'd have sex half the night and in the afternoon and before dinner." She laughs. "I don't know what the issue was. Maybe it was the rain. That was a happy time. I was very thin; I weighed about 120 then. The girls knew there was something going on. They were in eighth and sixth grade by then. I'd say to Randy, 'I'm going to take a nap. Do you feel like taking a nap?'"

Their sexual maturity, she says, allowed them to savor such encounters.

"We were older and more relaxed, and we could pack a week's worth of pleasure into an evening. I had multiple orgasms then. We used to get up [after lovemaking] and have cheese and crackers and orange juice—and 45 minutes later it was like a new night. We have had a very good sex life, up until the last decade. It was a gradual decline."

In 1993, Dianne quit smoking and gained 20 pounds. Though she eventually lost most of it, perimenopause brought another weight gain she couldn't shed.

"That's when my libido died and I sort of fell apart emotionally. It becomes a vicious cycle."

She remembers how after her girls were born, she'd occasionally tell Randy she wasn't in the mood for sex because she had "dishpan heart," which to her meant she was distracted by chores and couldn't think past the dirty dishes in the sink.

Over the years—and after their decade of delight—her disinterest in sex morphed into what she labeled a "black heart," and she would tell the persistent Randy that if he could banish her black heart, she'd have sex with him.

Randy worked hard to rekindle her desire.

"He'd look for something positive he could build on," she recalls, "like he'd rub my back and make me relax and then sneak around to some other place. And I'd say, 'My heart is still black.' So he'd try something else. And 99 percent of the time he'd erase my black heart. He could erase my excuses."

Dr. Whelihan applauds this scenario, even Dianne's honesty in communicating her lack of desire to her husband. She notes that if Dianne puts off intercourse until she's truly ready, her chances for orgasm are much better, and their (eventual) success rate gives her husband incentive to devise a way around her objections.

"He's called on to exercise all the seduction skills he possesses," Dr. Whelihan says. "And with persistence by both parties, their goal is met."

In 1997, with menopause further suffocating her desire, Dianne visited her former gynecologist, who prescribed plant estrogens. (She had yet to meet Dr. Whelihan.) They did nothing for her, but she developed a blood clot in her chest, so doctors advised against estrogen supplements of any kind. She took blood thinners for 18 months, then tried the soy route and several other homeopathic remedies.

"Nothing I took helped. I used to cry all the time because I just missed it. Sex was part of us. This was like a death in our family. We loved each other and that was the intimacy that kept us alive. It's part of sharing your inner self, your soul.

"You're so vulnerable at that time," she continues. "It's a giant trust and pleasure. You're giving each other a gift. I think of it more spiritually, even though the physical aspects are what drive you."

Through Cristina Ferrare's book *Okay, So I Don't Have a Headache*, Dianne found out about testosterone's ability to increase desire in women, but she was unable to obtain a prescription.

"[Cristina] uses a topical application of some concoction containing testosterone when she wants to get aroused. My doctor had never heard of it, of course. He said, 'Get me the recipe and I'll write it for you.' But how could I get the recipe?" Dianne asks. "I cried. I asked the next gynecologist I had, and my family doctor too. Of course, they were all men. They never heard of testosterone increasing female desire. They just told me about the detrimental effects.

"I know I'm not the only one," she continues. "Not that that makes it any better. A lot of my friends are in the same boat for one reason or another. Mainly the women don't talk about it, but the guys do when we get together. They'll say, 'Give her another glass of wine; maybe I'll get lucky tonight.' Some of my friends just say, 'That's past.' I hope it's not past for me, but of course it's been a long dry spell."

Dry spells are a fact of life for many women in their sixties.

"Estrogen and testosterone are produced by the ovaries, but at menopause, both disappear," Dr. Whelihan reminds us. "Among other benefits, estrogen and testosterone stimulate libido, so their loss can impact sexual desire. Many studies have looked at both safety and efficacy when using testosterone in women. Unfortunately, to date, there are no FDA-approved testosterone products for women, but many physicians, myself included, are comfortable prescribing it off-label with adequate supervision and consent."

With her libido already in shambles, in 2008 Dianne suddenly developed breathing issues, which began during a sexual encounter.

"I couldn't catch my breath. I thought it was because I got in that [passion] zone and couldn't catch my breath. But it became bothersome. After I went through lung function tests, I found I had reversible pulmonary disease. There's nothing wrong structurally, but it's like a giant asthma attack. It can happen out on the street, so I have an emergency inhaler. It's very, very frightening. And now it's part of the sexual issue."

These days, Dianne says intimacy is almost beyond her.

"Now I don't have the patience. I can start out with good intentions, but then my body goes, 'Aagh.' Sweat pours off me. [My husband] is very good. He regroups and sometimes we try again.

"If we get to the point where you're starting to sort of climb that mountain, and as long as I can stay calm and not have that air issue . . . once I'm aroused it's okay, but you can't dilly-dally. I climax quickly; it can be in three minutes."

Dianne gives Randy enormous credit for his skill and understanding.

"He's a very excellent lover; he's so patient and will try anything to make it good for me and encourage me," she says. "He's never sarcastic and he's never ostracized me. He knows how much I miss it. It's a major loss to him too."

When she and Randy do manage intercourse, she almost always achieves orgasm.

"But it's not like it used to be. It weighs heavy on me that

I'm not very reciprocating. My friends say, 'Just hurry up and get it over with.'"

But with zero libido, Dianne finds it difficult to say yes.

Dr. Mo says women with multiple health problems can still find help, even when passion is lacking. She prescribes testosterone for some of her patients, and though it does increase sexy thoughts, the motivation must still come from the individual, she points out.

"Sometimes you have to work on mood before you can address sex," she says. "Sex therapy can help. It's important to ensure the patient has balanced moods before we can address the issues with sexual desire."

Despite her statement about enjoying sex more in her sixties than ever before, Jana—unlike Dianne—can't point to a time in her marriage when her desire was particularly high.

"I just don't bring a large amount of sexual desire to the table."

As newlyweds, she and Mike had sex every other day, which leveled off to twice a week. It was when the couple resumed their love life after the birth of their first child that she experienced her first orgasm.

"I didn't know what [orgasm] was until I just had one," she says, clarifying that he was on top.

During most of their married life, Jana estimates she had orgasms about half the time; these days she's up to 95 percent. And often, she comes twice, which only began happening in the past couple of years.

The retired high school and college math teacher attributes this success to her being on top more often; she's just found that works well.

"It's the pressure on the clitoris when I'm on top that causes it," she guesses. "They're maybe two minutes apart. You say, 'That was great.' Then, wow, it's coming again.'"

The couple now has sex once a week, on Fridays, "since Viagra is so expensive—$18 a pill," says Jana. But too often, she arrives at the house at the last minute for their 4 o'clock date, straight from an errand or meeting.

"It's awful when I don't remember," she laments. "I feel bad, but that's the way I am. I don't want to take the time to do it necessarily, but once we get into it, I'm very interested. If it were up to me, it would be put off for a few days. . . . thank God it's not up to me. Mike will make sure we'll do what we're supposed to do."

Jana shares that Mike likes oral sex, so that's now always part of their routine.

"The oral sex lubricates the penis," she says, "and perhaps I am not so lubricated [since menopause]. So the mouth juices help. It seems to be what he wants; it doesn't turn me on but it's not a turnoff. I'm used to it."

As for her attitude about receiving oral sex, Jana says it makes her uncomfortable at first, but then she gets aroused.

"I still feel as if this is unclean. Not on my part, but his. What would he be doing in my vagina? It just feels unclean. But it is arousing, although it's not something I would seek."

Jana's husband has been using Viagra for three years, and she says that it causes him to ejaculate quickly. (But Dr. Whelihan notes that this is *not* a typical side effect of the drug: "Perhaps since he is getting a better erection and blood flow, he is having increased sensation and therefore it feels 'too good, too fast,'" she suggests.)

In any case, the result for Jana isn't ideal: "There isn't the fulfillment because once he has an orgasm, the penis relaxes;

it's harder for me [to finish]."

Her newfound ability to orgasm repeatedly causes Jana to reconsider the disinterest of her early married years. She wonders whether the decreased stress and worry of retirement have had a positive impact on her sex drive.

"I often regret when we were younger that we didn't explore these things. But we didn't. There were too many things to do. We had three boys. My mind was on other things all the time."

RELINQUISHING GIRLISH FANTASIES

Jana's regret is understandable, but like Dianne, she doesn't express disappointment in her choice of a partner. Of the rest of our spokeswomen, only Kay—who has been with her partner, Ann, for five years—is free of regrets and a degree of resignation.

Though she had four male lovers and perhaps 35 or 40 female lovers, she doesn't look back on any of those connections with bitterness and disappointment.

"Sex with men is not repugnant to me," Kay shares. "I just couldn't connect to a man to where I could love him and be with him and have a home and family with him. It was always a woman I felt that way about."

All the other sixties women who agreed to in-depth questioning display varying degrees of disenchantment with the male species, and appear to seesaw between a) wistful wonderings about what part of past failures belong on their own doorstep and b) realistic questioning about whether they even want new partners if they could find them.

"I think our society produces more women who are capable of healthy relationships than it does men," says our (former) California girl Laura, who was married for seven years in her twenties and whose last relationship ended eight years ago.

"Maybe it's a maturity issue. I'm attracted to men I hope I can fix. I know I can't, but I do it anyway. I have a lot of wonderful single girlfriends, and this is a common issue for all of us."

She tries to view her history with objectivity.

"Realistically if I haven't married in 40 years, I don't see it happening in my future. I'm happier being by myself than in a relationship because I get obsessive about everything, especially the sex."

WHY THE FOCUS ON FELLATIO?

Everyone knows men of all ages enjoy blow jobs. But the single women we interviewed in their sixties let us know that the guys they're dating seem more focused on oral sex than ever.

Laura, who divorced in her late twenties and is now 68, is rebelling against the increasing demands she fields for oral sex.

"I resent a man who wants oral sex more than he wants regular sex, because it doesn't do anything for me sexually. If that's what he wants more than anything, then he's selfish. I find as they get older, they want that more and more."

Dr. Whelihan explains that as people age, our sensory functions decline—throughout the body.

"In both men and women, increased stimulation is required to achieve the same results that were easier in the past. For men, oral sex provides both a heightened physical sensation *and* a visual turn-on. Together, they produce a more intense arousal, which helps men with dwindling erectile function."

"If that's true, then I'll just pass," Laura remarks. "I don't want to spend my life doing that all the time. I'd get really sick of [oral sex]."

It's not that Laura objects to giving blow jobs, just the frequency with which they're being requested.

"The last guy I was with, he was obsessed with oral sex. He had himself convinced that women get off just on that. Some do, I guess, but I can't do it for a long time. I don't think I've ever been with a man who didn't pressure me for more oral sex."

Sophia, a widow of 70, agrees with Laura: Giving blow jobs to her husband turned her off, and he eventually quit asking. But her recent boyfriend insisted.

"Today, I don't think men want sex," she says. "They just want blow jobs, I swear."

Laura's use of Paxil—for anxieties that she says are increasing with age—suppresses her sex drive. Still, she seesaws between her love of independence and her desire for a partner.

"On one hand, I'm spoiled. I inherited some money last year and I'm using it to remodel my house. I don't have to ask a man's opinion of what to do. I know what I want and I'm doing it. On the other hand, I recognize that I've never really had a partner in life. I do think that's the ultimate relationship and obviously very important. My shrink is on me about this. And I don't want to think I'm not going to know that before I die. But at the same time, every time I get involved with a man, he's so much trouble. I think I don't want to go through the trouble."

Jackie, the woman who says she's had enough of teaching men about sex, is also reviewing her history to see what lessons it might hold.

"Every man I've ever really cared about has cheated, so I have to look at myself and ask, 'Why do I choose that?'" she says. "I need to figure it out. Maybe it's the excitement [they offer]."

Leigh, our young widow, says that although she's had seven wonderful lovers in her life—the last one 18 months ago—she wonders whether perhaps her dating days are over.

"I don't know where to meet men anymore," she says quietly. "In my heart, I say I've been single too long."

DANCING WITH DESIRE

With her most recent lover, Leigh blames the relationship's demise on bad timing. But medical issues for both parties definitely figured in as well.

"I was his first relationship after his wife died. He wanted [to slot] me into the role of his wife. He was wonderful and I adored him, but he had a great marriage for 48 years and . . . you set patterns. I'm extremely independent after being single for so many years. He wanted to take care of me. I told him, 'It's a nice concept, but I have to walk beside you, not behind you.' I finally told him I don't think this is going to get easier. It was a hard thing to do, because I left really caring about him. He was very good to me. But I couldn't be what I couldn't be. I wasn't going to play that role. It would have blown up."

Sexually, their relationship required adjustments.

"I had no orgasms with him," she says. "He could get hard but he could not ejaculate. He kept getting upset, but I said, 'We're not messy; it's okay!'"

Leigh takes Celexa to treat hot flashes, which diminishes her sex drive. She's gone off it a time or two during relationships, but didn't in this case, since she felt it "evened out" their sexual desire.

Her relationship with the widower, who was three years older than her, lasted a little over a year.

Leigh says she once used a vibrator to achieve orgasm most

every night when she wasn't in a relationship, but now her frequency is down to once every four to six weeks.

"And it's not as strong a release either," she adds. "It was always hard for me to orgasm at my best. I cannot reach orgasm with a man through sexual intercourse. I can get close! For me, it takes manipulation with fingers or a vibrator or orally. I think it's the way the clitoris is positioned. Mine is maybe introverted [sic]. I don't know what they call it. It's hard for it to come out. It needs a lot of work. And I can't get it through sexual intercourse."

Leigh knows some men view simultaneous orgasms with their partner as the ultimate goal.

"That's the stigma in their head: We have to come together. I'm always honest, and tell them it's not going to happen. If that's what you need, it's not going to work."

The lively Leigh made ballroom dancing the social center of her life for a decade.

"It was a wonderful, passionate time of my life," she says of those 10 years.

She's says she's gone both ways in her dating, choosing one lover 16 years her junior and another 22 years her senior.

"I was always asking [my young lover] why he was with me. I'll never forget, we were having breakfast one day and I said something about masturbating. He said, 'See, *that's* why. You don't find that. No one my age would say that.'"

As for her older lover, whom she dated for almost five years, Leigh says friends couldn't grasp the concept of a 54-year-old woman being interested in a 76-year-old man.

"People don't understand what a wonderful lover he was. I met him through ballroom; we danced four or five nights a week. Once he got me into bed . . . he *knew* a woman's body. That was the key. He was patient and loving. The man was amazing. He taught me so much. It wasn't acrobatics; it was the entire body . . . slow and massaging. It was a total-body experience besides a sexual experience. And together it was beautiful. Younger men have this harder drive, but he was just slow and sensual."

Leigh makes an interesting distinction between married sex and single sex, calling it "an apples-to-oranges comparison. The married sixties I know are bored," she says. "It's the exception if you're not.

"When I was married, I was so tired that sex was not my first interest. If my husband initiated—which he always did, because I could roll over and sleep—once we got started, then I was fine. But honestly, I think most of my [married] friends could just walk away from it. We have to teach men, because there are very few men who know [to be sensual]. It's so easy for them; their goal is just to ejaculate. They don't need the foreplay. A woman, it doesn't work the same, for the most part. But if a man is loving, then he'll learn."

Though her marriage provided adventuresome and satisfying sex, Leigh says her first relationship as a widow opened her eyes to what she had missed.

"The intensity was much greater," she admits, "but it's not a fair comparison. I was married before; it was more exciting having my boyfriend over for the weekend with the kids gone."

Clearly, something about having sex available 24/7 renders it less desirable for many women. But the reality of waning estrogen, the side effects of drugs and the diminished availability of functioning partners all surface as complaints about sex for women in their sixties.

"As I'm getting older, sex is changing," Leigh recaps.

"WE'RE DOWN TO MUTUAL MASTURBATION"

Trudy, who suffered such guilt following her first sexual experience, counts about a dozen lovers since. After a breakup and two years apart from the man she cites on her survey as providing the best sex of her life, they are back together.

"He doesn't wine and dine me," she relates, and they split because "he just burned my butt and would piss me off beyond belief, because he essentially just wants a booty call." He still won't come to her family gatherings and doesn't invite her to his, but their chemistry overcomes all those differences.

"I gave up expecting more," says Trudy, a nurse care manager whose third marriage ended eight years ago. "I know he really cares about me. If that's all he can give, I can either accept it or not."

During the couple's breakup, Trudy didn't meet anyone else she liked, so when Johnny eventually called, she couldn't resist.

"I decided I might as well have sex! If I meet somebody, I'm going to go for it."

Meanwhile, Trudy sings Johnny's praises.

"He's older than me by seven years, but when we met, he was like a 45-year-old. He just rocked my socks. I've always liked sex, but it keeps getting better, so I figure the next one is really going to blow my mind."

Johnny's attention to foreplay, his interest in her satisfaction and his willingness to try anything make him a winner in bed. And though his prostate was removed due to cancer after they reconciled, Trudy isn't heartbroken that they are "down to mutual masturbation," as she says.

"Every now and then he'll get a slight erection, but it's not usable. But it doesn't matter. We know each other so well; we know all the buttons to push. He still loves to get together to touch and feel and hug and sleep after. He still likes to make love to me."

This surprised Trudy, whose third ex—when diagnosed with prostate cancer—almost immediately "just quit trying; he didn't want anything to do with sex. I thought he was having an affair." Instead, she found he had become obsessed with online pornography.

Dr. Whelihan believes "down to mutual masturbation" is a misnomer. Instead, she suggests we view this as simply the next stage, one that occurs naturally with age.

"Remember," the doc says, "men can climax with a soft penis, which gives pleasure to him, even though he can't penetrate her. Provided he does adequate clitoral stimulation, mutual masturbation is a viable and underrecognized option for those who are aging or have medical complications."

Johnny visits Trudy one to three times a week, depending on her work schedule.

"When I first met him, I could have an orgasm upside down, on top, missionary, you name it. Everything about him was just so sensual and stimulating."

Since her partner's surgery, she continues to climax with him all the time, saying she has "amazing orgasms" she never dreamed about. "I've even had G-spot ejaculations."

Whatever Trudy wants in bed is fine with Johnny.

"He has none of those worries about whether it's digital or oral or whatever," she says approvingly. "If he can't get me off with his cock, he could care less. He's a giving, giving lover. He doesn't let ego get in the way. It's all pleasurable for him, too. And he's not in a rush to have an orgasm either. Maybe that's an age thing. A quickie for him is about an hour."

Nevertheless, she occasionally looks back fondly. G-spot ejaculations in particular were more satisfactory before

Johnny's surgery.

"It was better if he could do it with everything working; there's a certain vibration in the cervix and uterus that you don't get with a finger that you do with a penis," she says. Sex isn't quite as exciting as it was in the beginning, she admits, but she remains extremely satisfied.

"I always felt like I was relatively uninhibited—not promiscuous, but uninhibited when I had a partner. With Johnny, I was the most uninhibited I'd been in my life. I could jump up and down on the bed if I wanted. Even with his prostate removed, because of the fabulous love we've made with each other, we're still friends. In fact, he wanted to see me more after he was diagnosed. It felt like what he needed was that touch and caring . . . more comfort, maybe. I'm not sure I care [about erections] that much anymore. I'm enjoying this so much. It's lovely to be held in his arms and touched. . . . It's the oddest relationship I've ever had."

THEN AND NOW

Newlywed Kylie and Sophia, our 70-year-old widow who recalls "Wild Is the Wind" fondly, also speak to the shifts age brings to a woman's sex life.

"I don't think I've ever found the man who is my ideal sexual partner," Kylie ruminates. "But he's in my head. In some ways, my present husband comes closest to it—but now that we're aged, he has his own issues. Not that that's a horrible thing; it doesn't bother me that you take a Viagra, but it can't be as spontaneous as it was.

"Sex changes," she continues. "You accept that this is what sex is like at this age. Which is not to say it's not good. You've learned all these things over your life. . . . At 20 there's this great,

'Ohhh, he's so wonderful; I love him so much' feeling, but I wasn't having great orgasms at 20. And I am now. It's too bad you can't combine the two."

Kylie's sexual history allows her to note, "Younger [men] are good because they have great endurance. And if you're out there [dating] for just the sex, you don't want an old guy who can't get it up."

Today, a content newlywed, she observes, "When you marry, you do lose your autonomy. I think my husband is a wonderful man. . . . And even though you love them you're coming from a different life experience. It's not that groupie kind of love, that rock-star adoration."

Kylie overcame that level of adoration when her first husband made a pitch to swap wives with a friend married to a woman with large breasts.

"That was the final straw. I realized this man did not love me. But I also lost a certain innocence you can never recover," she says. "I can't have the fairy tale. I hate that I'm not that person anymore. I liked that Kylie. I feel like I'm more hardened, more pessimistic. I'm more of a realist now, and it's probably a good thing I became that way. You don't look at the world the same anymore."

Sophia, who counts just three lovers in her life—one before her 38-year marriage and one after—compares her late husband to her postmarriage lover.

"Deep penetration with him on top," was her quickest route to orgasm with her husband, Victor, who was more generously endowed than either of her other lovers—thus enabling him to "stretch her out" and hit her clitoris.

"I call it the scissor position," she explains. "You can look at each other, see each other and touch in private areas that you can't normally reach."

Nevertheless, Sophia holds few memories of earth-shattering orgasms.

"It's a lie that [orgasm] sends you to the moon," she proclaims. "That's bullshit. It only sent me to the moon a few times."

Sophia figures she had orgasms about 40 percent of the time, and was married for seven months before she experienced her first intense orgasm, "where I went, 'This is great!'"

With Steve, who's now also deceased, Sophia describes a situation where sex seemed more of a commodity than it was during her marriage.

"I'm not saying my husband wasn't a good lover, because he was," she stresses. "He knew me. But Steve knew what turned a woman on, period. He really did. Within two minutes he could have me going. All those women [in his past] taught him plenty."

So did she have orgasms with him?

"Not many, but only because it took so long for him to get an erection, and then sometimes he couldn't complete [the act] because of his drinking. He'd get very frustrated with himself, and so he left me in a state of crap.

"But he sure knew how and where to touch," she offers. "It was like a discovery. Keep in mind this was a four-time-married guy. He knew every nook and cranny and where to go when he went below."

That said, Sophia couldn't help being repulsed by his crassness.

"He always sat with his legs apart. [Sometimes] he'd take my hand and put it between his legs and say, 'Get it going.'

"We could be driving down the street and he'd have his hand in my crotch at the red light," she complains. "We were more subtle than that when I was married."

Sophia fondly remembers many nights in bed with Victor when they would play strip poker as a variation on foreplay.

"He'd put on his socks and tie and underwear; I'd put on two pair of underwear because it makes the game go longer. We were good for at least an hour that way."

WHERE SATISFACTION LIES

It's not surprising, then, to discover that our sixties women have regrets and a certain degree of disillusionment attached to their lifetime of relationships with men. This is the decade when poor choice in partners or a stifling marriage can come back to haunt a woman's drive and function.

Sixty-somethings live without the naiveté of their youth, and are familiar with the concept of compromise, though they also mention the comfort to be found in less idealistic relationships.

None of the women interviewed in depth is currently seeing more than one person. In addition, as mentioned previously, not all are in sexual relationships. Laura hasn't taken a lover in seven years, Sophia in three and Leigh has been partnerless for 18 months. Of the married ladies, Dianne hasn't had sex in seven months, and for Kay and partner Ann, it's been a year and a half.

"We had sex every day and night when we first got together." Kay laughs. "I think I have a stronger sex drive than Ann. . . . As we got into the relationship, I realized she was pretty depressed. And now I'm taking antidepressants too, which has tempered my sex drive. I do feel better and more positive . . . but I guess you kind of get into a rut [sexually]."

The couple's lack of sexual intimacy—they've been together almost five years—doesn't particularly concern Kay.

"I tell Ann if I never have sex with her again, I'd still be in love with her. That's just one expression of how I feel about her.

Many of the women I know who have been together 45 years are not having passionate sex. What's binding them together is their love for each other."

As to her current situation, Kay says she would never go out and find someone else for a sexual encounter: "If I get to feeling really horny, I just masturbate."

Trudy, who has her visiting boyfriend, Johnny, and newly-wed Kylie say they have sex one to three times a week. Jana and her husband, who had sex twice a week for decades, are down to once a week, citing Viagra's cost as the reason.

Another interviewee, Jackie, never lacks for dates, but was between boyfriends when we spoke. Her frequency rate varied from a couple of times a week with her second husband to three times a day with her first.

I assumed Jackie meant that early in her first marriage they'd had sex three times daily, but she quickly set me straight. The couple actually *coupled* thrice daily for decades. It's no wonder Jackie could recite for me that their union lasted "20 years, 4 months and 20 days."

"I felt like nothing more than a receptacle. He wanted it first thing in the morning, last thing at night and at some point during the day. He'd come home at lunch for quickies."

There were no breaks she could recall—not for pregnancies, not for child care, not for anything.

"He was a good lover," she concedes. "A good kisser and good at foreplay. He was more technical than anything else. He learned where all my zones were and used them."

Jackie had orgasms about 15 percent of the time during their marriage, and says her practice of fantasizing during sex has its roots in those years.

"He wasn't happy unless he thought I climaxed too, so I

got very good at faking it . . . but I also think [fantasizing] was a defense mechanism to endure sex that frequently. I had four children; I was exhausted!"

Her adaptability was taxed greatly in that first relationship, yet Jackie went on to have many satisfying sexual encounters after their divorce.

In fact, she's in the minority of our 60-somethings in saying she *initiated* anal sex with one of her partners. It happened just once, with her second husband.

"It was at my instigation; it wasn't something that turned him on," she relates. "I tried anal sex with my first husband a few times, but it was just too painful [to complete]. It was a huge deal to my first husband, so even though my second husband was much larger, I think I wanted to share that with him. And it was good. . . . He went slower."

More than half our sixties interviewees had tried anal sex, so I asked Trudy, who was the most enthusiastic, to make a case for why she deemed this variation worth exploring.

"I know a lot of people find it to be frightening, but if you have the right partner and can relax, it's okay. I think part of the appeal of anal is there's a certain stimulus in that area. I can't explain it exactly; there are nerves there . . . and *if* the man is caring and gentle, you can relax those muscles, and if you go slow and slow and *slow* and you talk to each other, you could get to a place where you could have anal sex just as wildly as vaginal sex."

Trudy notes that she wasn't always so open, "but as I get older, if it feels good, I'm willing to try it."

Kay adds the secondhand perspective of some homosexual friends: "I've had a lot of gay men tell me that where their prostate gland is, it's very sensitive and pleasurable. So maybe they think it's pleasurable for women."

But Kay has never tried it.

"You touch-a my butt, I break-a your hand," she jokes, explaining that in college she had a fissure in her rectum that required surgery. To this day, she dislikes the presence of even a finger there during her routine gynecological exams.

"There's such a push [for anal sex] in our society," she observes. "I wonder if men aren't demanding it because it's dehumanizing."

Leigh, who avidly read all those books as a newlywed, believes a satisfying sex life doesn't require anal sex—though her much older lover made repeated requests.

"He begged me for anal sex, but I said, 'You can stand on your head, but I won't do that.' He used to say, 'I'll get you there yet,' but he didn't."

Sophia, who never consented to her husband's advances in that area, says simply: "I don't go that route."

Cunnilingus, however, is popular with all the 60-somethings I spoke with, though only two—Dianne and Leigh—named it as their "quickest route to orgasm." (Decade-wide, 26 percent of our 193 sixties women say clitoral stimulation is their surest way, with another 21 percent naming oral stimulation specifically.) For our interviewees, the most frequent answer is digital stimulation, while Jana and Sophia name penetration as their quickest route.

THE BEST EVER

As for the age at which women in their sixties had their best sex . . . that's a free-for-all. Trudy's having it now, with her tall, dark and handsome lover; Jana, 68, says now is her best time as well. For Laura it was during her early sixties: "I feel freer as I get older," she explains.

Kay says her best sex was at 50, when she hooked up with a 24-year-old woman with few inhibitions. "We had a great time, even though she was way too young," Kay relates. "I guess because I knew it wasn't going anywhere, I felt free with her. We explored different positions and types of stimulation. We were just all over the place—floor, bed, every room in the house."

For Dianne it was that "decade of delight" in her thirties, and Sophia, 70, was also happiest sexually during her thirties, specifically recalling a vacation escapade on the porch of an abandoned farmhouse one pitch-black night. Her husband talked her into a spontaneous detour during an ice-cream run for their daughters; Sophia still laughs about how the girls complained how mushy their frozen treat was when Mom and Dad finally returned.

For Kylie, a relationship she began in her late forties with a man seven years younger constituted her best sex.

"He was a self-described bad boy and he was always ready," she recalls. "He was sexual constantly, all day long. He exuded sexuality and kinkiness. He would have sex with me in unusual places, outdoors, in the boat, in the backyard, in the car. The fact that he was so animalistic about it, that's what turned me on. He taught me how much fun sex could be."

Jackie—she of the insatiable first husband—and Leigh—the ballroom dancer—both said they had too many excellent partners to choose just one. Lucky girls.

Perhaps not coincidentally, both women give evidence of libidos that require only minimal prompting.

Leigh's survey notes that she loses patience with partners who ask if she's "in the mood."

"All you need to do with me is foreplay and most times I'm

ready to go."

And Jackie's description of just her most recent "best sex" partner involves several encounters with Tim, 51, a man 13 years her junior. More than once, when she's dressed to go out for the evening, Tim arrives to pick her up, is turned on as soon as he sees her and the couple has sex on the sofa before they even leave the house.

A LIFETIME OF LIBIDO

Trudy and Kylie also mention the role their active sex drives have played in their lives.

"I'm probably an oddball about that because most women I know, if they're pissed off at their husband, they wouldn't even consider sex," Trudy muses. "I was probably bizarre. If he would seduce me, even if I were mad, next thing you know he'd have me laughing and the next thing you know we'd be in bed. I was softhearted. If you like sex, that's part of it. If [a man] wants to hug me, kiss me on the back of the neck, give me a few luscious kisses—I'm done, I'm Jell-O."

Trudy knows friends who withhold sex to get what they want, but says for her that would be like cutting off her nose to spite her face.

"Or maybe I just like the attention. When you're having sex, someone's totally focused on you." She laughs.

Kylie recalls zeroing in on her sensitivity to sensation, even as a young woman.

"I'm very tactile," she says. "I used to lie in my backyard stark naked in my twenties to get a tan. I would concentrate on the sun on my body and the heat of it and how it would make parts of my body feel. I would think about the wind and how it felt when it blew over me. I fine-tuned the nerve endings in my skin. I've tried to tell men [about this sensitivity], but they don't pick up on it."

The previously mentioned "animalistic" boyfriend, however, satisfied the more lustful aspects of her sexuality.

"I would be in the kitchen cooking and he'd come in and pull my shorts down and start giving me oral sex or just screw me from the rear," Kylie says. "You kind of look forward to it after a while. But also he'd just sometimes come into a room and push my head down [to his crotch], or point and demand oral sex. But I was willing. It wasn't demeaning. I knew it was going to turn into something fantastic. He'd give me what I wanted, so I was happy giving him what he wanted."

THE NATURE OF DESIRE

When asked about what creates and sustains desire over a lifetime, several women mention a difference they've noticed between the sexes.

"I think my attraction to the other person is what has affected my sex drive the most," surmises Trudy. "Which is always curious to me. Men don't have to have a focus on a particular person [to feel desire]. They can see a pretty woman and want to have sex with her. I try to explain this to Johnny. I don't want to have sex with a guy who's in great shape, say. I can feel slightly lustful about him, sure, but it wouldn't go anywhere unless I had an attraction to the person."

Leigh has a slightly different take: "Chemistry is what sustains desire," she says, "but it's chemistry for *you*. It doesn't have to make sense to anyone else. Three people can look at one man and all feel differently. I had a five-year relationship with this guy, and my girlfriend used to say, 'Tell me he's sweet, tell me he's kind, tell me any of that, but *don't* tell me he's good-looking.'"

Leigh's man was rugged and she admits he had a big nose, but "I thought he was the cat's meow. When you have that great sexual intimacy, you look at that person differently."

Kay addresses both the general and specific aspects of desire for herself, first touching on why she's attracted to women, and then how it focuses on Ann.

"Women's bodies are softer, they're not as hairy and they usually smell better," she explains. "I like the ebb and flow of sex with a woman . . . it's so intertwined. I don't know; I just prefer it! I guess I could choose not to ever sleep with a woman, but I know I would still be more attracted to women than men— because that's what I am."

What sustains Kay's desire for Ann is that she continues to see her partner as attractive.

"I don't know if everyone feels the same way, but when I'm in love with someone and they're my partner, they're the best-looking, most sexy person in the world. That doesn't mean I wouldn't acknowledge that someone over here is good-looking, but it's that, 'If I have sex, you're the one I want to have it with.' For me, it's the emotional bond I have with the person. Yes, we've both put on weight and we're going to Weight Watchers and all, but I look at her and she's the woman I fell in love with; she always will be."

DECADES OF DESIRE: THE SEVENTIES

Perhaps more than any other decade, the women we met in their seventies defied expectation. Bringing preconceived notions to the table isn't my style, but even so, Veronica and Gina, both 75, managed to surprise—and for opposite reasons.

Married for 48 years, Veronica was far from loyal to her husband and maintained a constant stream of affairs and sexual encounters, eventually racking up a lifetime number of lovers somewhat shy of 100. Within weeks of being widowed in 2008 at age 72, she had several trysts with a 27-year-old lover and then began a torrid affair with Juan, a man 30 years her junior who reignited the passion she says languished in the previous decade. Nevertheless, she's now trying to end that relationship, having discovered Juan to be both alcoholic and bipolar.

Gina, a doll-like blonde who doesn't look near her age, reports that back when she was 19, she and her boyfriend weren't able to achieve complete penetration for two full years after they first began having sex.

"The pain was just so bad," she recalls.

Nowadays, her history of sexual experimentation is behind her and she's happy to have physical intimacy relegated to the past. After a hysterectomy around 1982, she says sex with her second husband dwindled.

"He has trouble maintaining an erection; he tried Viagra once, but I told him it was bad for his heart."

"So . . . you don't want him to have an erection?" I ask.

"Certainly not! Where would he put it?" she replies with spirit. "You reach a certain age where everything dries up. Dry mouth, dry eyes, dry nose, dry skin . . . you name it."

Once you adjust to the charms of the unvarnished truth, the certainty of 70-something women becomes refreshing. For instance, even when wrestling with the core issue of her sexual desire, Nedia, 73, is delightfully outspoken.

"I think since I started going to this new church that I lost the desire to be sexy," says the tanned, bejeweled widow. "I don't want to go out and look for guys and have the affairs I used to. It's against my spirituality. I think I've gone holy. I still like to talk dirty and read a dirty book. And I don't think masturbation is a sin. . . . Didn't they give us that feeling for a reason? I do think it'd be a sin to be sleeping around, but I don't want to get married again, so . . ." She trails off with a giggle and a shrug of her shoulders.

Women in their seventies today were 20-somethings during the tumultuous decade of the 1960s, but the women interviewed for this book watched its changes unfold from the sidelines, so to speak. All our subjects were married and raising children—save for Gina, who's childless—during this time period, so their ability to jump in and experiment was limited.

Still, they were young enough to soak up the country's changing attitudes and the subsequent loosening of strict conservative mores. Sooner or later, two-thirds of the 70-something women I interviewed sought divorce, some more than once.

(Eighties ladies didn't end their marriages in high numbers; only one woman interviewed in that decade was a divorcée, although another remarried her husband after a year of divorce. In addition, 66 percent of eighties women had just one or two lovers; only 33 percent of the seventies women had that few.)

Within each decade, of course, are examples of long-term commitment and contentment, but in this age group, there's no missing the high count for divorces.

Twice-divorced Nedia is now a recent widow; her third husband died earlier this year. Twice-divorced Tori, who married her first love at age 18, is single today, and at 72 despairs of meeting an appropriate mate. Gina escaped an abusive first marriage after 12 years, and is now content with her practically sexless second marriage.

Each woman experienced a period of sexual experimentation and sampling between marriages, and each says she had between eight and ten lovers in her lifetime.

More conventional marriages are described by two other interviewees: Elizabeth, 73, and Sarah, who just turned 80. Both women married at age 19 and had satisfying sex lives with their sole partners, though neither woman is now sexually active. Both would like to be, but their partners' health issues make it impossible.

Previously mentioned Veronica was also married twice. Though at 35 she seriously considered divorcing her second husband to marry a younger lover, she changed her mind for financial reasons and went on to live a sexually adventurous life.

The women interviewed in-depth in this decade all had sex for the first time between the ages of 17 and 20; the average age was 18½. And aside from Veronica, they do not have particularly high numbers of lovers: Gina counts eight, Tori had 10 and

Nedia says eight or nine.

The theme of domestic violence—while mentioned in several age groups—appears most notably in this chapter, with half the interviewees rather nonchalantly describing incidents of physical or emotional abuse. This is double the one-in-four-women estimate given by the National Coalition Against Domestic Violence, and it seems probable that the economic dependency of women in this era was a contributing factor.

Not surprisingly, such behavior by an intimate partner has a profoundly negative effect on a woman's sexual desire, regardless of her age.

THE BIG PICTURE

Our total group of 70-somethings—118 women in this decade completed the survey—reveals a bit more about this generation of women.

Not a single respondent in this decade says the stresses of the day fill her mind when she's having sex; instead, 40 percent say they are either in the moment and feeling good, or just clearing their mind and staying blank. (Only the teens rate higher than the seventies women in this percentage!) Another 9 percent are thinking about pleasing their partner or making the experience better. And 13 percent are wondering whether they will have an orgasm.

True to form, 72 percent of women in this decade say clitoral stimulation of some sort is their quickest route to orgasm, with 23 percent of those specifying oral sex. Five percent say they rarely or never orgasm.

The most common answer for 70-something women when given the chance to name one thing they wish their partner would not do was, "Nothing; he's great." Since 21 percent of women in this decade wrote something to this effect, it could be a signal that with age, women learn to be satisfied with what they have. Or perhaps, with an open-ended question, if a participant can't think of a ready answer, she may default to something obvious—even if not strictly true.

WHAT 70s LADIES DON'T WANT

ANAL SEX	16%
RUSH TO INTERCOURSE	15%
BEING INSENSITIVE TO MY NEEDS	9%
TALKING DIRTY	8%
TRYING TO FORCE ORAL SEX	5%

Our spokeswomen for this decade weren't fans of anal sex; most of them had been asked, but only Veronica had ever experimented this way, and it was with her recent lover, Juan.

Kissing stimulates desire for almost 30 percent of 70-somethings, with touching named by another 12 percent. Closeness and cuddling work for 8 percent, and feeling loved is paramount for 10 percent of women in their seventies. Interestingly, almost 20 percent of women in this decade mention erotic videos, sexy books or porn as stimulants.

As for the best sex of their life, 12 percent say they are still waiting for it, but the rest are spread out fairly evenly between the twenties and the fifties, with the forties having a slight edge at 16 percent. Only two women in their seventies say they are having the best sex of their lives right now.

BEST SEX AT 70(?)(!)

We're all about good sex here at *Kiss and Tell*, so to validate the experience of women in their seventies having great sex, I wanted to interview one of the two ladies this age who wrote that she was having the best sex of her life right now.

Which is how I came to meet Veronica, a retired teacher from New York whose amorous adventures required a return visit for a second interview in order to faithfully chronicle her journey. As readers may recall, Veronica had perhaps 100 lovers, most during her 48-year marriage.

From the beginning, she says, foreign men attracted her: Her first affair was with an Italian waiter she met on a cruise with her husband, while her most recent lover, Juan, is a Dominican man. Their three-year relationship, which Veronica was struggling to end at the time of our interview, began four months after her husband, Gabe, died from the effects of a stroke.

"I was still in mourning. I wasn't looking for anyone," she says, recalling her first encounter with Juan, whom she met at a political dinner. Both had been drinking, she says, and when Juan kissed her good night as she left the event, her knees almost collapsed.

From the first time he made the two-hour drive from Miami to visit her, Veronica was hooked.

"He was the most amazing lover I'd ever had . . . the best of the best. When we had sex [the first time], I thought I probably killed him. I was so crazed and out of my head because I'd gone so long [without] and it was so good. I found out things about myself I didn't know . . . the sexual things he did that excited me. I just had so many orgasms it was unbelievable. He was great. I would scream."

As their relationship stretched into weeks and months, Veronica noticed unexpected changes in her postmeno-pausal self.

"My body started reacting—I began to have hot flashes

again, and my skin got very smooth."

With Juan, she's discovered she can orgasm during inter-course—a first for her—as well as have multiple orgasms during one session. She also shares that Juan discovered her G-spot when positioned behind her during sex.

But their lovemaking sessions have carried undesirable consequences as well.

"I've had black and blue marks inside my thighs; he's very rough," she says. "When he would turn me over, he would pull me by my legs. He's big, and when he thrust too hard, I would get a deep pain that felt like a bladder infection. That would happen very often. I would tell him he's too rough, but it didn't make any difference to him."

The two had sex at least once or twice a week, she says, and if he stayed over, it would be more.

"He might wake me up in the middle of the night. He was very sexual."

Now that she recognizes his bipolar disorder and has come to see how obsessive Juan is, Veronica is trying to end their rela-tionship.

"We fell in love almost immediately." She sighs in regret. "Or was it in lust? I can't tell the difference to this day."

A summation of her history indicates that Veronica did wander freely between love and lust throughout her life. She last tried to total up her lovers during her forties; she remembers counting "way over 50 men I'd had sex with."

She lost her virginity at 20 to a man eight years older, did a bit of sampling and then entered an eight-month marriage. After her divorce, another sampling period ensued, and then she married Gabe, a fellow teacher, in 1960.

She began her six-year affair with the Italian waiter—Peter—

in 1965, by which time she was 29 and had two daughters. She also was miserable. Not to mention sad and angry to find herself a stay-at-home mom—both bored and boring.

"Gabe was tired all the time and the girls had to be quiet," she recalls. "Here I was the party girl and I didn't even have a life!"

She resented Gabe's coldness and frequent absences while he worked two, sometimes three jobs. So Peter, whom she later learned was 18, became her first affair.

"Peter was a good lover, but not terribly experienced," she remembers. "I think I taught him more than he taught me. He was very loving and caring, a very sweet man, not rough. And he was better than Gabe; Gabe was a terrible lover. He was very fast. . . . He couldn't keep me coming long enough. And he would not initiate with me. I remember a lot of nights I would cry."

Veronica and Gabe had sex perhaps once a month, she recalls; meanwhile, when Peter's ship was in port, they continued their affair. Peter left the cruise line in 1970, when Veronica asked her husband to move out and her lover to move in. Her daughters loved Peter and he loved them, she says. The couple set a date to be married.

But at the last minute, Veronica had an epiphany.

"I woke up one day and said, 'What are you doing? This man wants another baby; he doesn't make enough money. But your husband is well situated, he could take care of the girls.'"

She nixed the wedding plans, and Peter went back to his former girlfriend, marrying quickly so he could stay in America. Meanwhile, Veronica called Gabe.

"I told him, 'Don't go to get a divorce; let's talk.'"

Gabe moved back in and the couple went to counseling, but Veronica says it really didn't help.

"Our marriage was not good. I did love him, because he took care of me and encouraged me to do things. But he was more like a brother than a husband."

So Veronica turned to a union president, a field rep, a tennis coach, a musician and others for more husbandly activities—always with a preference for foreign men.

"They love to kiss and show affection," the opposite of her husband, she says. "But they're just the fill-ins. I'm a basic person. When Gabe and I were separated that time, I didn't have the stability I would normally have. That stability was instilled in me as a child. I needed financial stability; I needed to know a man was there that I could trust."

Describing the evolution of sexual desire throughout her lifetime, Veronica sheds some light on her penchant for extramarital affairs.

"I wasn't single that long; I married at 22 and again at 24. So sex was exciting at first, but I didn't know much about it, and neither did the guys I was with. Gabe knew a little more than most, so that helped. I think when I started having affairs, that's when it got more exciting for me. The fear of getting caught heightened the excitement."

Despite her series of lovers, Veronica says she "wasn't a terribly sexual person."

"I only did it because it was comforting to me. I'm not a loose person. I won't go home with someone unless I just have to have him. But having someone [sexually] was taking the place of what I didn't have in my marriage."

During her forties, when her girls were grown and "didn't need their mother," Veronica experienced a phase she refers to as her "wilding" time. She describes it this way:

"That's when I was hot to trot . . . in my forties. I thought it was a terrible time in my life. I was happy when I was dancing at the clubs and going to the beach and being out and about, but I was angry and upset the rest of the time. We were constantly having parties and such. Gabe gave me a lot of space and I think that's the only reason I stayed. I met some guys in the Hamptons when we took a place there for a year. I used to go dancing three or four times a week at the clubs. Gabe wanted me to go. He'd say, 'Go dance!'

"I'd meet a lot of guys. I didn't have sex with them all, but knew a lot of people. I felt like I was out of control sexually in my head . . . not so much physically, because I wasn't doing that much. But I thought, 'I need help. This is not a real way of living. It's not healthy to constantly be looking for fun, trying to fill your life.' It was like I had ADHD. I needed to have all this fun and pleasure. I didn't want to be left out of anything. And we weren't."

Veronica—the only 70-something interviewee we spoke with who'd tried a threesome—recalls that it took place during this time with her husband and a girlfriend.

"She was divorced and I wanted her to have some pleasure. I was giving him to her. Afterward, I couldn't look at her. It wasn't that I was jealous. It just nauseated me for some reason. I couldn't figure it out. It seemed the right thing to do at the time, but not in hindsight."

Affairs always felt okay to Veronica until she detected a hint of the relationship becoming serious.

"I love when somebody loves me, but I know that if I married anyone, the sex would be over. It wouldn't be as exciting anymore."

For the now-widowed Veronica, missing the husband she cheated on countless times isn't ironic. She notes that when they retired to Florida 15 years ago, she contentedly settled down at last.

"I didn't take a lover in Florida; I didn't want or need one. I'd been looking and looking for somewhere to fit in, and then . . . *there* it is. It's right here. It was also very intellectually stimulating, because I joined a women's group . . . we traveled everywhere together."

Gabe was busy too; he was happy when their daughters visited, and Veronica says the couple at last started to have a fun relationship.

"There wasn't any sex, but I loved him. He took care of me, pampered me . . . he treated me like a princess. I was very spoiled by him."

Four years after his death, Veronica has yet to adjust to the absence of her husband of almost five decades. Though she expresses no remorse for her life choices, it's clear that her path didn't lead to the peace and acceptance she craves.

"I hate being single. I hate it. I was really happy being married. I miss Gabe so much. We had a great life and now I'm alone. I've never been alone my whole life. It's hard," she says, choking back tears.

SEVENTY AND SINGLE

Indeed, based on our interviews, being single in your seventies—while common—is not a cause for celebration. Tori, a lively 72-year-old who divorced her second husband in 1986 and has had a few dates since ("no boyfriends"), says it would take a very special man to attract her interest today.

"There's nobody that meets my expectations," she admits. "I'm very independent. That's why I don't have a boyfriend. I've more or less turned off my sexual desire since I don't have a partner. It'd take a miracle. I don't want the involvement."

And yet . . . she can't help wishing.

"Guys don't know what they're missing. I'm fun! I'm very sensual and sexual—what a waste. I cook too! I always say, 'I'm good in the kitchen *and* in the bedroom.'"

At 18, Tori married her first lover, Adam, a 20-year-old man who'd already spent a bit of time in jail. They became sexually active about six months before marrying—and Tori was pregnant when they wed.

"He was gorgeous, an Adonis," she recalls. "Very cute. Cute worked. I hungered for him. I felt nowhere near pretty, so I was thrilled with his attention. He was a sweet talker, you know? He bought me flowers and had a convertible. He always said he hoped my goodness would rub off on him."

That didn't happen. Adam was physically abusive, and the young couple's marriage ended after just two years: Tori escaped with the baby, the clothes on her back and the baby's diapers and bottle.

"Mom told me if I didn't leave, she'd tell the doctor not to treat me anymore when I came in [after beatings]."

For seven years Tori dated around, but most men she met didn't want a child. She estimates she had sex with seven guys during this period, usually one-night stands.

Even so, she still "practiced orgasms." She credits her experiences masturbating with her frequent orgasms when she does have partner sex.

"I knew my body and liked my body—and liked the sensation."

She doesn't remember masturbating after marrying her second husband, Keith, whom she stayed with for 21 years. She estimates that they had sex once a week, and reports that she had orgasms all the time.

"I was on top, always," she says. "I demanded it."

Tori told us on her survey that cute guys, sexy movies and her own lubrication stimulated her desire. For the "biggest lie" question, she says it was being told that women didn't climax as often as men: "I never had a problem, ever! I never faked one."

These days, her quickest route to orgasm is her fingers, and she masturbates a couple of times a month. If her fellow interviewee Nedia could give her a piece of advice, Tori would soon be hearing about the wonders of Waterpik to assist with that particular pleasure.

WATER WORKS

Nedia, also twice divorced like Tori, found a third man to marry—and they were together 33 years. Don died six months ago during heart surgery, and Nedia has no interest in marrying again.

"He was a saint; he's the only one who loved me unconditionally," says the deeply-tanned and fast-talking Nedia, though Don was a long way from being her best lover. After an animated recounting of a sexual history that began at 17 and encompassed eight or nine partners, Nedia confirms she's down to a party of one these days.

"My best orgasm now is with a Waterpik in the shower. They have a vibrating cycle. I can use my hand too, if I'm reading a book in bed. I used to have vibrators, but I threw them all out when I moved down to Florida 10 years ago. I taught all the girls in my Al-Anon group how to have orgasms with their Waterpiks and how to masturbate. They called me Dr. Ruth!"

Nedia, noting that there were times in her life when she "overdrank," says attendance at her new church has sharply curtailed her desire to be sexy.

She marvels at the change and seems resigned to her Water-pik (but is intensely interested to hear vibrator recommendations). She's candid about the days when she sampled her share of the real thing, and reveals a pattern of not leaving one man until she has another in the wings.

So she takes us back to the beginning—and says it all started with a lie. In order to escape her father's controlling influence ("I had an old-fashioned, greaseball Italian dad who wouldn't let me wear fingernail polish or lipstick"), she decided to get out from under him the only way she knew: She claimed to be pregnant.

Hardly original, but she *was* only 17.

And she was eager to have her own place, even if her 18-year-old boyfriend wasn't causing her young heart to swoon. She says she didn't like sex at first and remembers that her boyfriend stank.

She's hazy about her first time: "I remember a hot thing on my leg, but I don't remember having complete intercourse . . . just his hot dick on my leg. I remember [later] we had a tiny little apartment and all we did was punch each other out for a year. We argued and hit each other a lot. I did get pregnant right away."

Nedia's father dragged her back to his house after a year; she says he couldn't bear to see her meager existence. But the next five years were difficult, as Nedia came to suspect her father was bipolar.

She managed a few dates and even a lover or two, but her father's influence was oppressive. "He would say, 'Everyone thinks you're a whore; you're divorced and no one will marry you.'"

Freed from her physically abusive marriage, but now dependent on an emotionally abusive father, Nedia didn't see an easy out. But along came Joe, Nedia's second husband, to prove her old man wrong.

Once she'd bedded Joe, Nedia thought she'd died and gone to heaven.

"I never really liked sex until Joe. I remember dating him and I thought I'd met God. I was crazy in love with him. He may not have been that good, but all he had to do was touch me and I'd feel like I was going to have an orgasm. He was probably the first one I had a good climax with. He was so handsome, very sexy."

Unfortunately, Joe wasn't a one-woman man.

"He scooped me up and off my feet; I got pregnant right away," Nedia relates. "When I was first married to him, I didn't think about anyone except him. But he was a womanizer; he went with anyone at all."

He was also suspicious, and accused Nedia of being pregnant with another man's child shortly before they married, causing her to consider leaving him.

Nedia had two children with Joe—both his!—and their marriage lasted 10 years. She describes their first three years together, before she discovered his cheating, as among her best ever, sexually.

"We had sex probably twice a week and I would have orgasms most of the time, especially [during vaginal sex] from behind, when he also would touch me with his hands [on her clitoris]. That was the time I had the best orgasms."

However, once Nedia realized Joe would never be faithful, she began a series of affairs herself.

"I just ran around waiting for someone to make me feel like he did," she admits. At around age 32, she met Bill, who "I liked sexually and every other way," but who didn't want to marry her because she had three children.

"At least he was honest," she says. "But I was heartbroken."

Nedia says she was drinking too much during this time, and when things finally came to a head with Joe, "it was a lousy end to a marriage.

"We never had a fight that I didn't try to hit him. I wasn't a nice woman. I would smack him. I wouldn't take a slap or abuse or anything; I'd punch him back. I wouldn't go in a corner and cry; I'd smack him back."

With Bill unwilling to step up, Nedia's attentions wandered to her divorce attorney, Don. Married for 20 years, he later told Nedia he almost never saw his wife without her clothes.

"She used to lift up her nightgown and they'd have quickies." Nedia laughs.

Nedia and Don eventually married, but not for five years. She continued dating other men while Don's divorce dragged out.

"Don was Catholic and kept going back; plus I kept hoping Bill would marry me, kids and all. Now I'm glad he didn't, because he was an alcoholic."

When she and Don finally married, Nedia introduced him to oral sex.

"He'd go down on me more than I'd go down on him," she relates. "He liked sex, period. He used to go crazy just looking at my boobs. Toward the end [of Don's life], I would get on top so I could work fast and get it over with. I looked like a sexpot but I wasn't crazy about it."

Though Nedia "wasn't deeply in love with Don; not like with my second husband," she never cheated on him, perhaps because of his generous, unconditional love.

"I gradually grew to love and respect him, but there was

not that sexual 'wow' factor. He didn't know a thing about sex. I had to teach him.

"I did think about Bill sometimes when we made love," she confesses.

STILL MARRIED . . . AFTER ALL THESE YEARS

In sharp contract to the stories of Nedia and Veronica, both Sarah and Elizabeth have just one lover. Both were virgins when they married at age 19, though each had fooled around with her husband before the big day.

Sarah married Bernie in 1950; Elizabeth married David in 1958. Neither could foresee the sexual revolution just ahead.

"I went straight from my parents' house to my husband's," says Elizabeth, whose thick, dark hair and modern cut belie her years. "I was not part of that singles scene as we think of it today. I bought into the big thing that you had to be a virgin when you got married. So I was a good girl, and I waited. My husband and I look back now and laugh and say how *stupid* we were."

Sarah could hardly wait to get married to have sex. They'd done "everything but," and though Bernie was five years older and sexually experienced, Sarah's first time was a letdown.

"First of all, it hurt," she says. "I couldn't believe it; there was blood all over the sheets. I probably expected more the first time. And then it was over very quickly. It was a disappointment. But he learned to last longer. He worked on that."

Both women enjoyed satisfying sex lives, and neither raised the common female complaint of their thoughts straying during sex. Elizabeth says she focused on sensations, rather than thoughts, during sex, while Sarah says she often fantasized about her husband—or other men—masturbating.

"It's sexy to me, anyway," Sarah says. "You can't come if

you're thinking about [everyday] stuff."

However, during the periods when the women had young children, both faced challenges keeping their sex lives fresh.

"Those years of intense child rearing get in the way of everything else," explains Elizabeth. "I had a career, two kids close together in age, a hardworking husband. . . . Our lives were hectic, exhausting. But then the kids grow and you have time to focus on your own needs.

"We loved when our kids were gone on vacations or whatever, and we had those chances to be alone. We'd go to bed, bring some wine in, order a pizza. We had fun. I have to say those were the good old days."

Sarah tells a similar story: "When the kids were little, I was so busy. I was exhausted. Still, when we'd go away [for vacations or business trips], that was a different story."

She estimates that she and Bernie had sex weekly when the kids were young, but says she initiated more often on trips.

"We worked together, so we'd go on nice trips and have a lot of sex then. One time we came to Florida with our youngest. I remember we had to go into the bathroom in this one-bedroom apartment to get away from her. She was banging on the door: 'When are you coming out?'"

Throughout their marriage, Sarah says Bernie mostly waited for her to initiate sex. "He was terrific, very considerate." She grins.

Sarah began masturbating early, at age 4 or 5. "I knew my body, and that helps a woman enjoy sex. A lot of women don't know how to have an orgasm and it's sad."

Her quickest route to orgasm was always on top.

"Foreplay didn't turn me on as much as penetration," she states. "Not that I didn't like it, but I was anxious for insertion.

He'd say, 'What can I do for you,' and I'd say, 'You can be inside me.' I loved being on top. At least 90 percent of the time when I was on top, I would have orgasms."

How about oral?

"I gave him oral sex, but I didn't care for him doing it to me. I let him, but it wasn't that stimulating to me."

Elizabeth, on the other hand, loved oral sex, naming it her quickest route to orgasm. In fact, she says her first orgasm occurred when David was giving her oral sex early in their marriage. For variety, the couple watched porn films of the era, which Elizabeth says were pretty gross. Hard-core didn't turn her on, but she liked some softer porn.

Which reminds her: "You know in *Out of Africa* where Robert Redford is reciting poetry to her and shampooing her hair? *That* is drop-dead sexy to me!"

Elizabeth says she and David still shower together, as they have for much of their marriage. They now have a walk-in shower and often wash each other's backs.

But it has been years since they had intercourse.

"He has a number of physical problems, including high blood pressure," Elizabeth explains slowly. "All of the wonderful pills that have been discovered, he has not been able to take. It's not worth the dangers. At this point, we're relegated to hand-holding, cuddling. Retirement means we're together 24/7, and we're very close. But active sex has long been gone. I suspect it's troubling to him—as to me—but not overwhelmingly so. We do still have affection and cuddling. He's a rather romantic guy."

Elizabeth says the couple has made a few attempts at sex in the last couple of years, but she guesses it's been a decade since actual intercourse. She later asks David for his estimate—and he says five years. "Maybe it's eight," she suggests, smiling.

As for mutual masturbation, Sarah says it's been a long while since that as well.

"It's been one thing after another physically getting in the way."

She occasionally masturbates and says she once used vibrators from time to time—but not now.

"A handheld shower massage works," she offers, proving that seventies ladies are passing the word.

Has she asked David for oral sex?

"It's been a while," she admits. "I could ask him. . . . I might. I guess it's a matter of aging, but [sex] kind of takes a backseat. It's a shame, but I think it does. Even though I'm blessed with good health, I'm arthritic, which does make it harder to move around."

Sarah's sex life has also been pushed to the back burner since Bernie started showing symptoms of Alzheimer's a year ago. Long-standing prostate issues compound the problem.

"We can't have intercourse now, but we can fool around," she says. "We do some touching. . . . It's hard to tell if he has an erection."

She notes with shy pride that they were active until he was 84 and she was 79—and it's clear she is grieving what she fears is the permanent loss of this expression of their love.

"I guess I'm in a slump," she admits. "I'm sad about his situation. . . . It's very difficult. I've come to terms with it. There's other stuff that's more important now."

Elizabeth, however, remains hopeful for a restoration of her intimate life with David: "I'm not giving up. And actually I don't think he is either. I think we'll find a way. It was a really good, positive part of our lives."

NEVER A FAN

Not every woman finds sexual activity a lifetime source of enjoyment. In fact, some women are a long way from that experience.

Gina, who says she's happy to be done with sex, offers an unvarnished look at a life lived outside the throes of sexual ecstasy.

In 1980, at age 45, she married for the second time. Dan, 55, was Gina's eighth lover—and she's fine with him being her last.

"I don't remember exactly when we quit having sex," she says, "but I had a hysterectomy [30 years ago], and after that, we just didn't do it."

Gina's teenage memories of sex give clues to her attitude about intimacy.

"My mom let me know she didn't like sex," says the puckish blonde. "I think she had sex twice in her life and hated it. I must have her genes. I wouldn't even wear a V-neck as a teen because it was exposing too much."

Her dislike of sex was present from the start. At 18, Gina met Ed, whom she married five years later. After a year of dating, they attempted sex but, as reported earlier, were unable to complete the act because Gina found sex painful, even "excruciating," which is why it took years for the couple to achieve penetration.

Dr. Whelihan offers some medical clarification here, noting that some women have what's called a flat pubic arch (with less than the average curve), and although that creates more pleasurable friction for the man during intercourse, it can cause pain for the woman.

"Vaginas, like penises, come in all shapes and sizes," she explains.

Although the relationship of the vaginal size to the average penis is just fine for most couples, extremes do occur in the normal population—i.e., a smaller vagina and a larger penis—and a painful mismatch can occur.

With a candid conversation at a gynecologist's office, recommendations can be made for estrogen creams, lubes and vaginal dilators to make a painful situation more pleasurable. If your doctor doesn't initiate the discussion, take the first step and demand some resolutions. If none are forthcoming, consult another physician who may be more open to the conversation.

Back in the early 1950s, Gina just muddled through her miserable foray into sexual initiation. She does recall making real efforts toward intercourse: "I would get wet, yes. I really loved him in those days. But I can't remember all the details."

At the time, the couple didn't supplement their sex life with activities such as oral sex.

"Oral sex, in those days . . . the thought of that was repulsive," says Gina. "I didn't really even know about it."

Apart from their sex life, Ed exhibited a fear of commitment along with disturbingly possessive instincts, and Gina broke off their relationship several times, dating other men. She eventually became serious with a man named Jerry, and when they had sex she found it less painful.

"I was 21 or 22 and broken in," she explains. "I don't remember anything exceptional about sex with him; it was just run-of-the-mill. I probably had orgasms, I guess. But mine were never like you read about—earth-shattering and rockets going off. For me it's one, two, three and it's over. If you're reading a novel, you'll always read about multiple orgasms. I think people are making this up."

Jerry and Gina became engaged, but five weeks before the wedding, Ed made a last-ditch effort to get her back—and was successful. They married when Gina was 23.

"Ed was abusive right away," she relates. "Life was hell. He was paying me back for breaking up with him. He asked me if I had sex with my fiancé and I said yes. I should have lied, but I told the truth. And he had to pay me back."

How often did they have sex?

"Whenever he raped me," she states flatly. "At least once a week. It was very distasteful to me, because he could sustain an erection forever. I think maybe it was a physical problem. He could keep one for well over an hour. From that point on, I had a distaste for it."

Their marriage endured for 12 years, but for Gina, the sex never got much better.

"I can't remember, because it's a part of my life I want to forget. I probably did have orgasms with him; I don't remember them. I'm sure I had them when we were dating, once the two years of pre-entry were over, but once we married, it wasn't so good."

Ed was abusive physically and mentally; Gina felt lucky to extricate herself when she did. Finally free at 35, she entered the singles scene of the 1970s.

"I wanted to date right away. The freedom was wonderful."

She had sex with four or five guys during her decade of dating—and experienced a change of heart regarding oral sex. Orgasms, she discovered, were easiest with a tongue on her clitoris.

"There were a couple of guys who did oral sex, not many," she says, though she does remember the partner who was the best.

For positions, she had a clear favorite: "I was always on top. When I was dating, that was the only way I could get an orgasm."

To a question about whether she recalls any time in her life when she had consistent, enjoyable sex, she cites the early days of dating Dan, her current husband.

"It was real good with him. There was nothing earth-shattering, nothing out of the way [as far as orgasms]. But it was enjoyable. I had finally met someone who was a really nice person, who was the total opposite of my first husband."

Gina says the couple had sex a few times a week until her hysterectomy a couple of years into their marriage. Toys, porn, sexy books and such were never part of their routine.

Though intercourse ceased after her operation, Gina says she will "relieve" Dan on special occasions—specifically during their frequent cruises—by giving him a hand job.

(Nedia mentioned a similar vacation arrangement with husband Don: "Every vacation we took, we'd have 3 o'clock sex daily. A little before 3 I'd be like, 'Shit, I gotta do this.' But oh, boy, he couldn't wait. He never forgot when it was time.")

BUTT NO

No woman interviewed for this chapter said she likes anal sex.

Nedia says she screamed at one of the married men she dated for trying it and said, "Forget it." Neither Sarah nor Tori had partners who ever brought up the idea, and neither woman wanted to try it.

"If [Dan] were to get it up, which he can't, it's like a wet noodle," says Gina. "But even if he were [hard], there's no way in this world he would want that."

"We talked about rectal penetration," says Elizabeth, "and to me that's just bizarre pain for no reason. Uh-uh. The subject may have come up and he may have suggested it. However, he would never force anything on me. We've used finger penetration, but not penile penetration. That's a major turnoff for me."

Which leaves Veronica. Though she had many lovers, she

says only one tried to force the issue—that is, until she met Juan. That first time, many years ago, she refused.

"Len [her lover] thought I was fooling around with his friend. He knew it was a place he shouldn't be and he wanted to take it. Of course I didn't let him. I've had anal sex with Juan only. I didn't know anybody else who wanted that, honestly."

Our survey indicates that younger men much more frequently show interest in anal sex, which may be why Veronica had so few requests before meeting Juan, who's 46. And despite her general euphoria about sex with Juan, she did write "insist on anal sex" as the one thing she wishes her partner would not do.

WHAT ENDURES: A LOOK BACK

Women in their seventies have a rich history on which to reflect, so it's worthwhile to ask them what building blocks sustain or just affect desire throughout a lifetime. Once again, their forthright answers bring some surprises.

Veronica says romance affects her sex drive the most, specifically a little wine and a nice dinner. But during her self-described "wilding" time, she says dissatisfaction with her life affected her sex drive most. "Having a man inside me, with me, beside me, holding me, whatever, that's what I craved."

Nedia says her weight affected her sex drive more than any other single thing.

"I was always overweight and didn't want anyone to see me naked. I think if I'd been thinner, I'd have been a big whore. But I was ashamed for anyone to see me. Ever since I was 13, I was on a diet."

Tori says no one thing affected her, but that she "felt a strong sexual desire all my life, ever since I was a teenager." She recalls her late years of high school as the time of her strongest urges. But at 72, she's "more or less turned off my sexual desire, since I don't have a partner."

For Sarah, verbal affirmation affected her sex drive the most: "His compliments—that's what kept me going all through the years."

However, she is moved to mention that her desire for Bernie increased after a midlife-crisis fling he had with another woman.

"My desire for him really was tremendous after I found out about the affair. I confronted him and I even threatened to leave, but I wouldn't have. He ended it willingly. It took me a while to get over it, because it's very hurtful. But I know he loved me. And he became so sexy to me after. Not right away, but certainly once I got used to it. I don't know why, but . . . oh, it's crazy! Who knows why?"

Gina's take on what affected her sex drive most significantly is perhaps predictable: "It was drying up and the pain factor." As for what sustains sexual desire? "I can't think of anything. I don't want it, so it's hard to give you an answer on that one. I don't want any part of it now. God forbid something happens to my husband; I don't think I'd even want to date. I have everything: my own side of the house, my dog, my master bedroom . . . everything I need is here."

For Elizabeth, still married to David after 53 years, desire seems to be about a certain type of solidarity.

"I guess it's a romantic approach, a love . . . wanting the warmth, the closeness, the intimacy," she says.

She and David went to a counselor when they were in their late fifties, which Elizabeth says was very successful in helping them understand and forgive the small irritations they felt.

"It pulled us together quite a bit. When you're together with someone for so long, you fall back and forget to work on things. Everything is taken for granted and it's very dangerous."

The counseling clarified for the couple that despite their transient complaints, neither had any desire to split up. And Elizabeth says their sex life improved correspondingly—until David's health issues developed.

To sustain desire, Elizabeth not surprisingly believes health and energy are essential, "because when you don't have it, it really gets in the way. If he had more energy, I think we'd be buzzing along. Our hearts are in it, but our bodies aren't."

In fact, despite all their frank and revealing talk, the majority of our interviewees have bodies that are no longer engaged in an active sex life, whether it's just been six months—in Nedia's case—or the previous 30 years, in Gina's.

Fortunately, these lively women seem to be nurturing their memories while trying to remain open to the possibility of future passion.

DECADES OF DESIRE:
THE EIGHTIES

Today's sex-soaked culture makes it hard to imagine what it was like for a woman to experience her sexual awakening in the 1940s. But that's when our eighties ladies began having sex, which for most wasn't until they had a ring on their finger.

The average age among this decade for first-time sex was 18, and in looking for commonalities, it's worth noting their interest in oral sex was quite low overall.

Because so few women of this era received sex talks from their parents—or even whispers from their friends—their first-time bedroom encounters held the potential to be quite a shock.

"The first time we had sex, I cried, just looking at his penis," says Rifki, an 85-year-old widow recalling her honeymoon. "Even though I had three brothers, I'd never seen it long or hard. And it was right close to me. I was afraid to go near it. That was stupid, my own fault. I should have gone to the library and read up. I'm sure my girlfriends did, though they never mentioned it."

Since many of the 52 women in their eighties who filled out our survey were restrained in their language, revealing few details as to the particulars of their love lives, it was a bit of a surprise to discover during our in-depth interviews that they were having or had enjoyed extremely satisfying and active sex lives decade after decade.

Once they warmed to the alien freedom of speaking openly about sex, they poured out information and details, occasionally getting fuzzy on a date or a name, but mostly able to recall as many particulars as anyone could hope for.

Overall, these senior women proved to be happy and satisfied with their sex lives, often praising their husbands for being patient and gentle in their early, inexperienced days, thus ensuring happy coupling for many years to come.

Rifki, who now lives in a seniors' community, says her husband didn't push her the first night or two of their marriage, in deference to her fears.

"He was very gentle, very considerate, and took it slow," she says. "I was very appreciative of that. Then once we started, oh boy. He taught me how to have orgasms. I would never have known if he hadn't. It didn't always go quickly with me and yet he was very patient."

Rifki's surest path to orgasm was oral sex, so that became a regular part of the couple's sex life.

"He would not enter until I had an orgasm," she remembers. "He was a very thoughtful person. He knew if I'm not fulfilled, then I'm not interested. [Sex] was always very pleasant. I always enjoyed it."

Rifki's comfort with oral sex—or even experience with it—is an anomaly among the eighties ladies who completed our survey. Overall, less than 6 percent of this age group say their quickest route to orgasm is oral sex, while their younger equivalents show substantially higher numbers: For instance, almost 26 percent of 30-something women say oral sex is their quickest route, and just over 20 percent of women in their sixties say the same.

Low interest in oral sex by no means keeps women in this age group from immensely satisfying sex lives. Sharon, 82, is a case in point.

At five-foot-six, with coiffed white hair, an elegant figure, earrings and makeup, Sharon looks at least 10 years younger than her age. Her first and only lover is Joseph, to whom she's been married for 61 years. She was 21 at the time of her marriage—but not a virgin.

"We had sex right off the bat," she says of Joseph. "I couldn't help it. He was unbelievable. He had a way of kissing . . . he devoured you. I've kissed other men, but oh, God. He's got these hot lips, even to this day. And he was gorgeous. He had a beautiful body, clean, smelled good."

A little prompting elicited the information that, to Sharon, "right off the bat" meant several months, and that Joseph's legendary kissing never includes any tongue.

"I don't like French kissing," she declares. "I think there was one guy that did it and I pushed him away and said, 'Don't ever try that again.' Joseph never did that. I didn't have to tell him anything. We were very compatible."

Though Sharon was eager to have sex, she too was uninformed.

"Nobody spoke about sex," she recalls. "Everything was a big secret. I think I was curious more than anything else. Even your friends didn't talk about it."

But Sharon is clearly enjoying the chance to recall her courting days, and goes on to describe her capitulation to Joseph: "We were talking and caressing; it was so nice. It felt good. The house was mine, because my mother and father had a luncheonette and were never home. When he came over one afternoon, I said,

'Oh, to hell with it.' I was a little shy, but he was very manly, very sexy. The kissing and hugging and talking and whatever; then sex became something I wanted. I knew [society said], 'Before marriage, how could you? Tsk, tsk. Shame on you, girl.' And then I thought, 'To hell with it.' At that time, you didn't have sex before marriage."

Like Rifki, Sharon says she found a patient, considerate partner.

"When you have a man who's tender and loving and knows how, that's the answer to [continued desire]," she says. "I wasn't hurt. He showed such caring. It was more important that I should feel good, not him. Even to this day, he never considers himself. How could you not love him?"

Joseph and Sharon walked down the aisle less than a year after their sex life began, and a tour through their wedding album reveals no fewer than three pictures of them kissing at the reception.

"Sexpot," says Sharon of her groom, with an air of satisfaction.

DAILY DELIGHT

Sharon's self-satisfaction is warranted. She describes an active sex life that, until her husband's recent prostate issues, included intercourse with simultaneous orgasms almost every day from the time she and Joseph became engaged. In their sixties, the frequency dropped to four times a week.

"If it could have been twice a day, we would have been twice a day." She laughs. "I just looked at him and that was it. He gave me a kiss. He still does that. He's hot stuff. He doesn't look it, but his sexuality is unbelievable. And how he used his hands!"

Though she enjoys Joseph's hands and lips, Sharon's orgasms occur only with penetration. (She notes that he's well-endowed.)

"If intercourse is better, why would I want anything else? I gave him oral sex once; I didn't like it," she says, though Joseph did. "I wouldn't like him to give it to me."

No one position works better than others for Sharon to reach orgasm. As for foreplay, not much is needed.

"I give him the sign: 'All right, let's go.' I'm more assertive than him," she states. "In fact, maybe I'm aggressive. Then when you get into bed, he's fondling and touching a little bit here and there. Five minutes [of foreplay] is enough."

A question to Dr. Whelihan concerning Sharon's ability to orgasm in multiple positions through penetration alone provides some insight:

"Most of the current literature reveals that 70 to 90 percent of women require direct clitoral stimulation to achieve orgasm. However, when you look at the 10 to 30 percent who indicate that they can climax with intercourse [penetration], 90 percent of *that* group specifically states they must be on top. That's because this position creates indirect clitoral stimulation, from the partner's abdomen or pubic bone. But if the penis is big enough, it may stretch what's called the 'legs' of the clitoris, which extend down under the labia major [or puffier lips]."

So in Sharon's case, size matters.

The couple's sex life began deteriorating in their mid-seventies; Joseph's gradually enlarging prostate caused a corresponding decline in his lovemaking abilities.

"It was so pathetic when he couldn't do it anymore," Sharon says. "It's like his manhood is gone. He tries to do everything else to compensate. But it's not the same."

Since the couple usually had orgasms together, Sharon is loath to have one without him, so she's attempted to convince Joseph they should try mutual masturbation. As a teenager,

Sharon engaged in masturbation, but she's been unsuccessful in convincing her husband of its pleasures.

"Joseph says he wants to take Viagra, but I say, 'No, you can have a heart attack.' He's been two years unable. I say, 'One of these days I'm going to get you into masturbating. You've got to open your mind to it.' He says no way in hell."

Dr. Whelihan acknowledges that there is much confusion regarding Viagra, a drug initially developed to treat angina (chest pain).

"In the early trials, men reported the unexpected and thrilling side effect of good erections," she says, "so Pfizer quickly switched tracks and developed Viagra as a drug for ED, or erectile dysfunction."

The reports of heart attack while on Viagra are minimal, and have more to do with generally unhealthy men who have been inactive for years "suddenly bouncing around the bedroom with their proud erection." It's the overexertion from the performance that causes ischemia (heart attack), *not* the Viagra, she explains.

A few drugs, such as the Nitro-Patch or nitroglycerine, cannot be used with Viagra, so it is contraindicated in these patients. "Otherwise it is a miracle drug for many men," the doctor says. "Ask your cardiologist, your urologist or a savvy primary doc and you will be amazed that the answer is likely, 'Yes, it's okay!'"

A SECOND CHANCE

Catherine, an 84-year-old newlywed of two years, is married to a Viagra user, though she notes that her husband, who's 77, doesn't need a pill every time they have sex.

"He asked me if I cared if he got Viagra and I said it didn't make any difference to me. He might use it from time to time, but he never makes an issue of it. At times, we're not expecting it [to have sex], like in the morning or something, so then he will not use it."

Catherine, who writes on her survey that she's having the best sex of her life "right now," is an inspiration, and her experience proves the adage that it's never too late to kick-start your sex life.

Raised by a housekeeper and a mom who traveled the world as a musician, Catherine was solitary, but not unhappy. She adored her much older brother, but never formed attachments to any of her mother's eight husbands.

She married at 15, to the first boy she dated, who was 18 and on his way to being a state patrolman. She adored him, she says, but didn't have sexual desire for him.

"My mother-in-law said sex was a wifely duty, so I probably looked on it as a chore that went with married life. It was part of being a wife. It's too bad. I realize now I didn't have the desires I probably should have. If you're told it's a duty, it isn't as much fun."

Catherine's husband told her sex was something you did to show your love.

"I was a child really," she recalls. "We had sex a couple of months before the wedding. I was pregnant when I got married and I didn't even know it. I was so dumb. No one thought to educate me. I thought the baby would be born through my navel. Everyone kept me in the dark."

As time passed, Catherine learned to live with her husband's alcoholism and his string of affairs.

"He made me feel used," she says. "I knew when he was fooling around—every time." The clues were there: He didn't want sex with Catherine when the affairs were going on, and afterward, he'd buy her flowers or presents.

"I don't think I ever really enjoyed sex during my first marriage, not really," she says sadly. "If it's something you've never had, you don't miss it. It's just not there."

In 1988, after decades of marriage, Catherine's husband died from cirrhosis of the liver. For 20 years, there was no one. She worked as an accountant and dated a handful of guys.

"I wouldn't go out more than once because then I'd have to go to bed with them," she says. "I thought they'd expect something. I've never felt at ease with men."

In 1999, Catherine moved to Palm Beach County and slid comfortably into retirement community living. For almost a decade, the pleasant, grandmotherly-looking lady played bingo, attended local events and stayed busy.

Then, during a party at the clubhouse, Catherine's daughter invited George to sit at their table. Catherine had seen George around the complex occasionally, had even known his wife before she died.

The party included dancing, and though she turned him down several times, George persisted. Finally her daughter grabbed Catherine's hand, placed it in George's and said, "She'd love to dance."

"I rarely dance with anybody, only my husband," reports Catherine. "But I couldn't believe it, I felt comfortable with him! I wasn't stiff as a board."

She went home early, "as I always did," but a day or two later George called and asked where she'd gone. They had their first date later that week, and something about his accepting manner changed everything.

They became engaged in April, but Catherine confesses shyly that she was "just a little bit worried about sex." Though everything felt brand-new with George, she couldn't help but be afraid that physical love might feel like a duty, as it had for 40 years with husband number one.

"I made up my mind that I wanted to go to bed with him before I got married," she states, as if this is both shameful and shocking. "I didn't want to feel pressured with it, that it wasn't going to be a duty. I didn't want an extra chore. That's putting it pretty bluntly.

"So I went to bed with him," she says.

Before the wedding. Just to make sure.

And it was wonderful, because at 82, Catherine had her first orgasm. But it was painful too, because her vaginal dryness was severe enough to cause bleeding.

"Even though it hurt like mad, I knew I had feelings I'd never had before," she recalls.

She didn't want George to know of her discomfort, so she went to talk things over with Dr. Whelihan.

"How long since you've had sex?" asked the doctor. When the surprising answer was 1988, Dr. Mo prescribed Estrace, an estradiol vaginal cream Catherine still uses weekly to treat the area.

The couple now enjoys sex on average once a week.

"I have sexual desire for George, which I really never did for my first husband," Catherine says. "I don't think I ever felt passionate before."

Life with George has brought other shifts as well.

"I've changed so much. I don't feel so uncomfortable with men. My first husband was very jealous. I was always afraid he'd get angry if he thought I was flirting. I had this feeling of always waiting for the other shoe to drop."

What stimulates her desire today?

"Maybe it's when he makes remarks that show he cares about me. Something he says will make me know I don't have to watch what I say. It's a good feeling, a feeling I never had before. And he teases me unmercifully. Oh, my gosh! It's wonderful. I don't have to be on guard. It makes me feel warm and makes me want him to hold me.

"Sometimes [in bed], George just holds me. Before, I knew it would lead to sex. I *knew* it. It doesn't always with George. I had never, ever instigated sex before, and sometimes I do with him. Once, he'd gone to bed early, and I was watching a show, a tearjerker. That aroused me. And I went into the bedroom and he was still awake waiting and was receptive. I instigated it!"

Catherine has orgasms about half the time she and George have sex. While oral sex isn't part of their routine, she's had orgasms with him on top or sideways and "occasionally with him just fooling around with his hands."

"A couple of times I have and he hasn't," she confides. "It's okay."

She indicates that George nurtures her desire, taking his time to get her in the mood.

"He doesn't just say, 'Let's go,'" Catherine explains. "I often tell him how I feel and I know he appreciates it. Usually I'm receptive to him. There's been a few times I just didn't feel like fooling around and he accepts it right away."

During our extended interview, Catherine never exhibits a "poor me" attitude, never questions the fates that kept her from an enjoyable sex life for so many decades. Only happiness and gratitude for her current good fortune are in evidence, so it's touching to watch her reiterate the answer to the survey question concerning the best sex of her life.

"It's right now," she affirms, "beginning at 82 with George.

It's been wonderful. I feel free and I feel whole. It's nice just waking up beside him every day."

The bonus? She didn't realize until they took out the marriage license that he was seven years younger than she is.

"I don't know why I didn't know how old he was," she says. "But now I call myself a cougar."

ANYTHING ELSE, BOSS?

Catherine found happiness with her second lover, Sharon and Rifki with their first, but not all women now in their eighties confined themselves to sex with their spouses. Victoria, a self-described "career girl" who didn't marry until 32, and Emma, a precocious learner who had perhaps 15 lovers between the ages of 16 and 22, provide glimpses of alternate routes to sexual fulfillment.

These adventurous 80-somethings are the minority, however; two-thirds of the women interviewed in this decade had just one or two lovers. Only one eighties lady had more than eight lifetime partners, while two-thirds of women in their seventies count that many lovers. And only a third of seventies women are still with their first partner, compared with half the eighties women who are still married or are widows who never took another lover.

Career girl Victoria, a just-turned-90 widow with perfect posture, gold jewelry and red nails and lipstick, describes a classic "affair with the boss" scenario, which began when she was 18 and lasted for 13 years.

Though her married boss, Jerome, was 25 years her senior and having a simultaneous affair with her fellow secretary, Victoria felt no resentment then or now.

"The other secretary? Sure, he had her too. I wasn't stupid," she says. "But this was in the '40s. A lot of things were different. I admired his genius and brilliance—he had eight degrees. He made me part of what I am today.

"I didn't feel I was taken advantage of. Maybe I was a little naive, but this was a totally stimulating new life. It was very glamorous. There was a car, plus a big salary of $10,000 a year, all the perks, meeting all the bigwigs. I was very absorbed by that. I was taken to all these beautiful places in New York, introduced to a new way of living. He wanted me to go to night college and I did. He opened a whole new life for me."

During their years together, Victoria had no other lovers.

"Promiscuous I wasn't," she says, though she was approached by many. "His other copresidents approached me, those sons of bitches. I was loyal to him."

Nevertheless, Victoria describes a fairly tepid sexual relationship, not a tempestuous affair.

"In retrospect, he was not a good lover. He was mundane. But I was a man pleaser; I didn't know any better.

"I had made him so powerful as an individual—he was *king*," she elaborates. "Not because of sex, but because of my whole personality. I was young and vibrant and I had the animal quality of a woman that age. I was a willing subject with him and he with me."

And yet: "I never thought of wanting to have sex with him. I never had an orgasm with him—and never realized it until I had one after that. I came down on him [oral sex], but he never came down on me. He should have given me what I wanted as a woman, pleased me to the hilt. But I didn't even know what it was."

Ask Victoria what stimulated her desire back then, and the only thing that comes to mind is "pleasing him."

"That was my persona for quite a while." And then: "I used to have a drink with him and it would stimulate me to let him come back to my apartment. It liberated me from thinking I was doing something wrong. It was my excuse to go."

A reversal of fortune landed her boss in jail, and Victoria moved home to the Bronx with her mother. She dated regularly, and attributes her continued fondness for much older, often married lovers to the fact that her father died when she was 8.

One suitor during this time, Vic, was a Chicago businessman, smitten with her and "married, of course." He sent orchids, perfume and gifts every day.

"He was a great lover," she remembers. "He educated me. I used to meet him at five o'clock in the morning when his plane came in. We shared some exciting times. I had my first orgasm with him; he was the first one who came down on me. He taught me about oral sex."

Around this time, in the early 1950s, Victoria recalls a period when she had three lovers at once: a policeman, a coworker and a third man whose name escapes her.

She describes a powerful sexual connection with the policeman, who was 12 years her senior and someone she dated for a year.

"He wasn't a potential suitor or partner; we had sex at hotels, and I didn't like the setup," she says. "I was too high-class for that. But the attraction was strong. It was the first and only time I had anal sex. I think I had an orgasm through the anal sex, too. I don't have any idea if that's common."

She can't recall whether during that encounter he stimulated her clitoris, just noting, "It was not my way of having sex. Maybe I thought it was dirty."

Victoria found her period of experimentation brought consequences.

"Three suitors," she says. "It was too much. I got cystitis. How much can my body take? It was a short interlude. And then when I met Morley, I went on the straight and narrow."

MARRIAGE—AT 32

Victoria met Morley on a 10-day cruise; he sat down next to her at breakfast. Before the cruise ended, the divorced attorney (who at 44 was 12 years her senior —surprise, surprise) told Victoria he was going to marry her.

And three months later he did.

He brought her to New York shortly after the cruise and arranged their first lovemaking experience.

"We stayed in a hotel and had continuous sex all day long," Victoria remembers. "Our chemistry was fantastic. He was a better lover and I got educated."

The couple soon had two children, and though Victoria always worked and life could be chaotic, she says the attraction never waned.

"It was always great. Either one of us could instigate it. I was not bashful. We had sex once a week, or once every two weeks—more frequently earlier in the marriage. Before my kids, he'd come home and I'd be in bed nude waiting for him. I was aggressive and wanted to be."

Once normalcy set in, Victoria admits her brain would sometimes wander during sex, and she might think about appointments for the next day. Eventually, about five years into the marriage, she realized she was disappointed by her husband's lack of aggression as a businessman, though she never let on.

The couple didn't experiment with anal sex and never employed gadgets, "sex pictures" or toys. Victoria says they didn't have to: "The chemistry was always there."

Even so, intercourse didn't produce orgasms for Victoria, even when she tried being on top. Oral sex was what worked, and she describes her first few years with her husband as the best sex of her life.

"When it was mutual it was the best—pleasing my husband and myself," she says. "In fact, I would get emotional and start to cry sometimes. Those first five years were the best."

The couple remained sexually active until the final year of Morley's life, when he became too ill. He passed away at age 74 and Victoria soon moved to Florida, where she discovered that the cancer that caused her to undergo a mastectomy in 1974 had returned. Shortly after her second mastectomy she met Robert, an accountant 10 years her senior, in a business setting. Not long after, he asked to take her out.

"I told him I just had a mastectomy and I was waiting for my prosthesis, and he said, 'Okay, call me.' I was so frightened. . . . I didn't know if I'd be attractive."

Friends asked Victoria what she saw in Robert, since he had no aggression or vitality, the hallmarks she had always looked for in men.

"I was way ahead of him, smarter than him," she says, "but he accepted me as a woman. It was sort of a survival attraction as a woman, you know what I mean?"

The two went together for 12 years, though Victoria discloses that she never experienced orgasms during their encounters.

"I taught him, you know what I mean? When I went down on him, he went crazy."

VIBRATORS—AT 80

When Robert had a stroke, it was Victoria who cared for him. After his death, she didn't immediately seek another lover.

Instead, at 80, she discovered sex toys.

"My girlfriend bought me a vibrator," she exclaims. "I thought it was terrific. I could have sex without a man! Since then, I've educated women, and they say, 'What? A vibrator? I'm too old.' They shrug. But then occasionally they come back later and bless me.

"You have to be careful who you talk to," she warns. "Some people think you're a sex maniac. But I'm liberated, through and through."

Victoria's most recent sexual partner was a neighbor in her complex, three years her junior.

It was several years ago, she says, and "he was too old to do anything, [i.e., intercourse]. I was free as a bird after Robert died and it was almost to see if I still could. It was a pattern. I became a man pleaser again."

She brought him to orgasm through oral sex, and he wanted to reciprocate, but she wouldn't allow it.

"He didn't have anything to offer me. He was the Lothario type, a son of a bitch. He sort of dropped me and went with someone else."

Without remorse, Victoria returned to her vibrator. Now 90, she says she is still orgasmic, but no longer has multiple orgasms, a talent she discovered when she first began using a vibrator.

"I'm not dry as a woman," she announces. "I'm attributing that to using the vibrator. People atrophy there and I'm not atrophied. I bring the blood down there and stimulate the area, because that can be very painful to be dry."

EARLY TO THE GAME

Emma, the previously mentioned precocious learner, was an

early adopter in many ways. She wasn't just intelligent, she also developed physically at a young age. By 10, she was a freshman in high school; by 11 she had menstrual cycles. Her breasts developed at 12, and by 14 she was allowed into clubs to drink, thanks to her lenient parents. She started college at 15, and sex wasn't far off.

Some of her memories of partners are fuzzy, and she admits her lifelong use of alcohol—she quit drinking four months prior to our interview—doesn't help her hindsight, but at 82, Emma does have sharp recall for some pivotal moments in her understanding of sex.

"I remember on the way to high school, there was a big Bloomingdale's between the bus and subway," she says. "I loved to cut through because their book department was on the first floor. I loved books; I was such a reader. I found a book there that was graphic, and it described the actual insertion. I remember standing there thinking, 'Oh! Is that it?' Other girls had been hinting and I never knew what they were talking about. I was used to being a smart kid, but I was also used to being the youngest."

Prior to her epiphany in Bloomie's, Emma was experimenting with the pleasurable sensations brought on by enemas.

"The enema bag and equipment were always in the bathroom, hanging on the wall," she says. "If any of us kids [she had three siblings] got constipated, Mom would give us enemas. At that age, the enema felt good. She'd say, 'Hold it in as long as you can,' and that's when it really felt good."

Dr. Whelihan notes that the early stages of development—which include oral (thumb-sucking as a soothing behavior) and anal (learning to control bowel movements during potty training)—are crucial in shaping our behavior as adults. How someone processes these early stages influences adult behavior and may find expression in a variety of ways.

Emma read the classics from a young age, and though she had no idea yet what sexual intercourse was, she remembers taking characters from books to construct sexual fantasies early on.

"I even wrote some of them down and would read them while giving myself enemas. One scenario involved David Copperfield getting punished by his cruel stepfather. In my fantasies, he punished David with an enema. It was always a punishment; I came up with that myself. Mom didn't punish us with enemas."

Emma describes carving old-fashioned soap suppositories into cone shapes, which she inserted rectally in ever-increasing sizes.

"I would choose a story and use them in order," she says. "After a year or two, I started just using the two largest."

With one bathroom in the house, Emma says she must have planned carefully to get time alone: "The other kids were very outdoorsy. It must have been when Mom went shopping or next door to my aunt's for afternoon tea. I know I didn't do it at night, because my bedroom was a flight up from the bathroom."

From age 14, Emma looked and acted older, so her world opened up early. She took it all in stride.

"We were nouveau riche by then," she says. "I considered my dad a playboy of the Western world. He took Mom to all the clubs, Broadway shows, opera, everywhere—and he'd take me because I could pass for older."

Emma adored her father, who she now realizes was alcoholic. He encouraged Emma to drink around this time, and she says she began smoking as well, a habit she kept for 64 years.

Her first lover—a man named Ed of an undetermined age—

came along when she was 16.

"We were in his car. . . . I'm sure I'd had a lot to drink. He kept pleading with me to let him put it in, and I kept saying no, I'd never done that. In my memory it just went in a little bit. But he seemed to be satisfied. He may have ejaculated. When I got home, I don't remember any come, but I did see a couple of drops of blood on my panties. From then on, there were a number of guys, but I don't know their names. I must have been drunk a lot of the time—but I was doing well in college."

She had orgasms right from the start: "Shortly after the penis was inserted, a few thrusts and I'd have an orgasm," she says. "If he could keep it up, I'd have another one a few minutes later. My desire for sex was very strong. It's difficult to separate how much of it was physical and how much was mental."

She had no girlfriends; instead she "wanted to be with guys and have sex all the time."

She met her husband at age 22, and estimates that by then she'd been with 10 to 15 partners, several of whom who were quite elderly.

"They weren't good lovers; I just got a kick out of the fact that I could play them for fools," she says. "I was so egotistical at the time. One guy took the bus to work with me—he must have been in his seventies. I had him just begging for more after I went off with him one time [for sex]. I just loved having someone beg me."

Once she was married, Emma's desire focused exclusively on her husband, Jim. She met the good-looking local soldier when he was on Christmas leave from Okinawa. She refused to have sex with him during his leave, wanting their first time to be special.

"I knew right away he was different," she says. "He was it for me. To this day, he was the love of my life."

She never cheated on Jim, though she was tempted. At parties, she might be stimulated by others, but couldn't wait to get home with her husband.

Jim was the first man Emma had anal sex with; she says she realized right away she loved it, although she didn't connect that pleasure with her childhood enemas until recently.

Like Emma, Jim was quite a drinker, "Probably alcoholic," she reflects. The couple had two children, but the marriage lasted only nine years. They drifted apart, and when she left him, Emma briefly moved back in with her folks, who had moved to Florida. She hadn't worked while married, but now returned to the academic life she loved, eventually earning master's and doctorate degrees while teaching school.

"This is when I started masturbation," she shares, though clitoral stimulation was not her preferred route.

"I found I could have an orgasm by having a bowel movement. Then I'd only pretend to have a bowel movement. It took only a few minutes. I'd either imagine a scene from a book, or use erotic literature I'd collected. I would feel it coming and put it off and put it off. When I had fantasies, I'd imagine myself as the rapist, not the victim."

Emma did date during this time, but when men wanted sex, she would say she just couldn't.

"Occasionally I would have orgasms just from kissing or from him pressing against me, and he would know that and say, 'Let's have sex.' I was physically ready, but not mentally, so I said no."

BACK IN THE GAME

Emma met Al around 1970, when both were in their forties, and the two were sexual partners—and once even housemates—for the next 30 years. Other than a two-year affair with a man 13 years her junior while working on her doctorate in north Florida, Al was her only lover for those decades.

Right from the start, Emma knew there was something different about Al's penis.

"It was bent at a strange angle, and it was always only semi-hard. I looked it up and it had a name: Peyronie's disease. I asked him about it one time. He hadn't heard of the disease and said it had always been like that. He didn't want to talk about it.

"As long as it got hard enough, I was okay," she summarizes. "But with Al's bent penis, I found that me on top was the best position."

Al also suffered from premature ejaculation, so Emma says she did a lot of masturbating. But she enjoyed giving him blow jobs, which was Al's preference anyway.

"In fact, that excited me and would give me an orgasm," she says, without simultaneous clitoral stimulation.

But she didn't enjoy being on the receiving end of oral sex and never experienced orgasm that way.

Between 60 and 70, Emma's sexual desire declined. She masturbated, or turned to Al for increasingly elusive satisfaction.

"I became more demanding of Al, because [sex] required more stimulation," she says, "but he was getting weaker. So it dwindled out of its own accord."

The couple last had sex a dozen years ago, and Emma reports that she hasn't felt any desire since about that time.

When asked about vibrators, she says she never had one and wouldn't get one now because she doesn't miss sex.

"I don't think about it anymore. But from 30 to 60, I was horny all the time."

A STRUGGLE TO REACH THE PEAK

A decline in libido isn't unusual as a woman ages, but some women in this decade struggled from the beginning to achieve satisfaction. When asked for their quickest route to orgasm, 7 percent of the 52 women in this decade who participated in our survey answered that they'd never had orgasms. Almost 9 percent left the question blank; one woman wrote that orgasms were rare for her. And another, the aforementioned Catherine, memorably had her first orgasm at 82.

These less-ecstatic expressions of sexual desire are certainly valid. Jane, an 82-year-old widow of nine years, affirmed in a phone call that she never experienced an orgasm, but enjoyed a loving relationship with her husband of 50 years.

Her mother warned her not to let boys touch her on dates, and Jane waited for her wedding night to have sex. She doesn't recall how her husband would let her know he was in the mood, but says he never asked her to try things she didn't want to try, including oral sex.

Clearly uncomfortable discussing such particulars about her sex life, she merely says, "We had a lot of love for each other and were the best of friends, besides."

Today, she says multiple medications prevent her from feeling desire for any kind of sex.

"When he died, my heart was broken. I haven't really looked for anyone else."

WHEN YOU LEAST EXPECT IT

Jane may not be looking, but other 80-somethings have found they don't need to look—love finds *them*. As is true for every age, where there are men, there are sexual invitations to the women around them.

Catherine certainly wasn't on the prowl for George, and Rifki, the first widow mentioned in this chapter, wasn't looking for a partner when she moved to her senior citizens' community. She'd been widowed for nine years and says she'd long since substituted a showerhead and warm water for the oral sex she once enjoyed so much with her husband, Elias.

But after just a few months in her new digs, Rifki met a widower, Kyle, down the hall who "decided he'd like to have sex with me."

How did this coupling come about?

"He invited me to his apartment. . . . He used to love to stretch out on his bed. And he invited me to lie near him. That's when it started. He started to undress me, so I asked, 'What are you doing?' And he said, 'You'll like what I'm doing.'"

The pair had sex twice a week for several months, but then Kyle was transferred to a nearby assisted-living building when his health deteriorated.

Rifki says Kyle has asked her to come visit, but her sciatica is acting up, and a walk across the vast lawn to his new room is daunting. Besides, it's not like it was with Elias. She doesn't have orgasms with Kyle, and she misses Elias's wooing ways.

"Elias was an English major. He would say such beautiful things that put me in the mood. Whereas with Kyle, it's, 'C'mon over here; lie down.' Very ordinary. So I felt Elias was the better lover."

There was one complaint about Elias that Rifki *was* willing to mention: "He put his tongue in my mouth while enjoying sex. I couldn't stand it." What bothered her about it? "The dampness, I guess."

Sex in your eighties holds its own challenges, and Rifki mentions one she's now facing with Kyle: "He's very skinny and his bones hurt as he climbs on top of me. They're sharp! And he's still losing weight. So I'm not rushing over to see him."

Rifki doesn't know if she is Kyle's only lover, but says, "Knowing him, he's tried with many women. Men enjoy having multiple partners, you know."

Yep. We know.

DECADES OF DESIRE:
THE NINETIES

MEET OUR OLDEST SURVEY RESPONDENTS—WOMEN IN THEIR tenth decade of living.

These are the women with the most years of experience and potentially the most to teach us about the ebb and flow of desire throughout a lifetime.

But be aware: These are also the women with the least practice at giving voice to their intimate desires. Their sexuality unfolded and matured during a long-gone era of restraint. It was a time when "virgin wedding bed" was more than a figure of speech; when conversations about sex—if they happened at all—took place almost exclusively between husbands and wives; when sex was extremely private, not the ubiquitous media presence it is today.

Several of the women in this age bracket were so reticent on the subject of sex that they turned down a face-to-face interview: They either didn't want to be overheard in their living facilities speaking with someone about sex or insisted that they couldn't offer enough information about their sex drive to make a visit worthwhile. In these cases, delicate telephone conversations elicited as much information as possible before the woman's level of discomfort caused her to—graciously, of course—bring the conversation to a close.

A few of our nineties ladies had faulty memories: In fact, one woman hung up after stating that she couldn't remember yesterday, much less intimate details about her long-dead husband. Nevertheless, considering the strictures of the era in which they were raised, some of the women were remarkably candid.

Consider these facts: No 90-something woman had received a sex talk from her parents, most had never talked about sex with a doctor and all had confined their sexual activity to their marriage partners. Each was a virgin on her wedding night; only one said she engaged in heavy petting the week before the ceremony.

It was a different time, and in deference to the sensibilities of its survivors, certain intimate questions were broached only when the candidate demonstrated that she was open to deeper interrogation.

One widow stated that in her marriage of almost 50 years, she and her husband had never tried oral sex. Another said she accepted the wedding proposal of her soldier boyfriend when they had exchanged chaste kisses only. One woman mimicked her parents' approach to sex education, saying that while raising three sons, neither she nor her husband felt it appropriate to initiate sex talks with their boys. To this day she doesn't feel bad about not giving them information.

When you compare this mind-set to our survey respondents in their twenties—roughly the age of their great-granddaughters—the distance between these generations seems vast. When asked to share the number of lovers she'd had, one 21-year-old interviewee said she lost count "somewhere in the 30s." Such a life path is all but incomprehensible to a woman in her nineties.

In contrast, the ladies in this decade come across as steadfast. They display simple loyalty to their virtues, to their cultural values and to their husbands.

SEX—YES OR NO?

If you skipped ahead to this chapter, overcome with morbid curiosity to discover whether women in their nineties are even *having* sex—and if so, how exactly they're accomplishing it, given their physical realities—you might be disappointed.

The truth is that of the 11 women in their nineties who filled out our survey, none are currently having sex. (Anecdotally, Dr. Whelihan knows of several women in their nineties who *are* active; they just didn't happen to participate in the survey.) While our interviewees have fond memories of their husbands as lovers, and often admit to missing sex with them, none are interested in new partners.

When pressed, no specific physical issues were cited that restricted these senior women from enjoying sex lives; rather, it was lack of interest and a partner.

In fact, survey-wide, senior women didn't often bring up their own physical limitations. Dr. Whelihan says this speaks to the fact that with appropriate stimulation—which activates dopamine release—and the right amount of passion, a woman's boundaries, both physical and emotional, usually melt away.

Lack of desire, not ability, was the most often cited reason for celibacy at this age.

"I'm not a sexy person," says Sue, a twice-widowed 91-year-old. "I loved both of my husbands, and sex was my way of showing love."

But as the years unwound, her desire dwindled. Before her second husband died—when Sue was in her eighties—the couple was having sex just five or six times a year. "That's plenty," she announces.

Sue is the only twice-married interviewee from our 90-something group—and she had no expectation of a second love until a divorcé in her retirement village actively pursued her.

All but one of the other interviewees in this age bracket are widows who count just one lover in their lifetime—their husband.

"Once is enough, honey," quips Katherine, a 94-year-old widow who married at 20 and stayed that way for more than 60 years.

She "absolutely" waited for her wedding night, and her husband was her only lover. "It's not like the kids today," she says. "They jump in and out of bed, and that's where the problems come."

Katherine, a widow for 30 years, says she no longer misses sex. "You learn to put things out of your mind," she explains.

Gwen, 98, also had a sole partner. A widow for 20 years, she enjoyed an active sex life with her husband, describing frequent orgasms and sex at least twice a week. She "definitely" misses sex with him, even after so long. "We were part of each other," she says of their bond.

But she has no desire for a husband now. A divorcé in his fifties showed interest in her a while back, but Gwen says she admonished him: "I'm not for you!"

Evelyn, also 98, was married for 66 years and didn't desire another lover after her husband's death 12 years ago.

"There are times I could have used a partner," she says, "but I didn't want anyone but him, only him, because we loved each other so dearly. Sure, I miss having sex with him, but not to a desire where I wanted to have it with anybody else."

Malka, a tiny, 92-year-old fireball, is the most articulate and plain-speaking woman of her decade. Her candor provides valuable insight into the plight of women her age who lose their partners.

A virgin when she married at 23, Malka enjoyed a lifelong attraction to Reuven, her husband of 41 years. Even on his deathbed, she recalls, "If he just reached out and touched my hand, it sent a thrill through me."

About a decade after Reuven died, Malka had a brief, months-long relationship with a "gentleman."

"I tried having sex with him two or three times, but I couldn't continue," she relates. "It wasn't fair to him, and I wasn't doing myself any good. I'd always made love with my husband and couldn't make love to [this new man]. That's the reason I never remarried. I never met a man that I could respond to physically like I did Reuven.

"And, of course," she says, "as you get older, there are less and less dates," referencing the frustration all aging women face.

Malka tried masturbation a few times after her husband died, but "it wasn't the same." And then it became painful.

"It hurt. I'm dry."

She says now her desire is "completely, 100 percent gone."

Dr. Whelihan says this is not unusual in women in their nineties.

"Since we understand that vaginal dryness begins with the loss of estrogen at menopause, realize that in their tenth decade, these women have been deprived of their estrogen for almost 40 years.

"Estrogen increases the elasticity, lubrication and plushness of vaginal tissue, and only those women on hormone therapy maintain its advantages."

The doctor notes that vaginal dryness tends to be a chronic, progressive problem unless treated with estrogen.

"Estrogen now comes in various forms, including pills, creams and a ring," she says. "We can treat only the vagina if a woman doesn't want to treat the whole body."

She notes that older women who continue using hormones into their nineties are true believers, staunchly insisting their continued health is due to that practice.

Though Dr. Whelihan still sees gynecological patients in this age group, once a woman passes 85, the risks for many cancers, such as cervical, breast and colon, is on the decline.

"At this age, the screening tests done by the gynecologist are unnecessary, because we're not so worried that they'll die of cancer. However, I find that my ladies in their nineties enjoy the social interaction of a visit. They love to hear how mentally and physically healthy they are from the doctor. And they are!"

DETAILS, DETAILS, DETAILS

For the majority of our 90-something ladies, sharing the details of their sexual history for this book constituted the most substantive conversation they'd had on the subject *in their lives.* Even spunky Malka, the only woman adventurous enough to have tried oral and even anal sex, was woefully uninformed on her wedding night, by today's standards.

"You have to understand, I had no one to talk to," she says. "I didn't even know about orgasms. He was very patient with me. . . . I didn't know how he entered exactly. I knew sperm entered the vagina, but I didn't really know how. I was learning everything new at one time."

Her husband, who'd had many lovers before her, knew she was supposed to have an orgasm, and Malka says he wasn't going to stop until she did.

"I was a wreck. [It took time], but I found when he stimulated the clitoris—with his finger or his penis—it was easiest. We had variety, but when I see what they're doing today [with some of the toys], I think, 'I wish my husband was alive so we could try that.' We were so repetitive. I didn't even know those things were around!"

Toys may not have been part of the repertoire, but other things were.

"We tried oral sex on each other," she says, with enjoyment on both sides. "As long as I had an orgasm, it was fine with me."

As for anal sex, Malka wonders whether the idea occurred to her husband at the beginning of their marriage. If it had, she thinks he would have given her an indication, because she says she was a willing partner to experimentation. "We did try it later on," she reveals, "but he knew that I didn't like it."

For Malka, sex "was exciting for all the years I lived with him." He was away for 17 months in the service, and, "It was not easy to have that pent-up sexual energy all that time. I never asked if he had any affairs then. If he'd said yes, I would have been destroyed. If he'd said no, I'd always have doubted it, because I knew what kind of man he was. He was a very sexual person. I responded well to him."

After an initial honeymoon period in which Malka says she often "couldn't wait" for sex, she and her husband settled into a routine of twice, sometimes three times a week.

"I imagine there were times when I felt I was too tired; I had four children! But he was the prime object of my life; my kids were secondary—and they knew it."

Malka remembers that "when he'd kiss me good-bye in the morning sometimes, I'd say to myself, 'He's gonna come back.'

It was because I knew he wouldn't be able to get through the day [without sex]."

Sure enough . . . he'd find an excuse to stop by later or come home for lunch—and more.

However, Malka declined to use the word *quickie* for such trysts.

"It was never a quickie. He didn't believe that I was worthy of a quickie," she explains. "That was what you did with all the girls you met around. With your wife, he believed you had an obligation to make sure she wanted it and enjoyed it."

Gwen, our widow of 20 years, recalls similar spontaneous encounters with her husband.

"After the kids were grown, he would show up at lunch sometimes, and I knew why he was coming," she says with a laugh. "It was a good marriage sexually. I was satisfied. We were compatible."

Gwen's memories are valid, but like several of her contemporaries, she seems to cast a rose-colored tint over her now-distant sex life. For instance, she professes never—in almost 60 years of marriage—to have had sex with her husband when she wasn't in the mood.

Evelyn also is unable to recollect any flaws in her late husband's technique. When asked for the one thing she wished he wouldn't do, she said it was hard to give an honest answer.

"To me, everything was so ideal. There probably was something I wish he wouldn't do, but I can't remember it. As far as my mind can remember, we always had a great sex life. Just being near him was enough to stimulate me. Anything he did, anything he wanted, was great for me."

Clearly an optimist, Evelyn later says, "I only think of the positive things in my life. I'm 98; I'm glad I remember my name!"

She does recall that she and her husband put effort into their sex life.

"Most of the time we both had orgasms; we worked at it until we both did. And when I say worked, well, you do have to work at it."

Evelyn shares that the couple normally had sex in the missionary position, but "there were other things we did before he reached that point."

She pauses. "I'm glad you're talking about it, because I love to think of him. He's with me all the time. I feel such gratitude for having been with him."

SECOND TIME AROUND

When women in their nineties are able to overcome their natural reticence, their stories provide insight into how drastically times—and sexual mores—have changed.

Though she was 23 on her first date with Jay—he asked her to a civic center dance where a big band was playing—Sue was still naive. She said Jay was a good dancer, but denies that dancing with him stimulated her.

"I wasn't thinking in those terms back then."

Jay left for service in World War II and wrote her throughout his tour of duty, eventually proposing by mail. The couple had kissed before he left, but nothing hot and heavy, Sue says.

What caused her to accept his proposal?

"I'm a Christian and he's a Christian, and he was a wonderful young man," she says. He was a good kisser, she shares, but doesn't recall whether that influenced her decision.

(Dr. Mo offers a timely observation here: "Both kissing and dancing initiate dopamine release, a stimulator of sexual desire.")

Sue married Jay when she was 25, but when she looks back,

she's unable to pinpoint any decade or time as being especially satisfying sexually. In fact, none of the women interviewed in this group could identify a time in her life when sex was best.

Sue does recall that Jay was very patient, "a gem." All he had to do was "love her" to stimulate her desire. When asked whether clitoral stimulation was her fastest route to orgasm, as she indicated on the survey, she merely nods.

None of her responses indicate an adventurous sex life; she politely answers, "Oh, no," to a query about trying oral sex. As for frequency, Sue estimates she and Jay had sex once a month.

"I wasn't ever a sex kitten."

She describes her second husband, whom she married in 1992, as a "touchy-feely guy." He died of cancer and was a "terrible smoker and drinker, which I knew, but he was a peachy guy anyway."

Their romance caught Sue by surprise.

"When Jay died, it wasn't in my thoughts at all to marry again. It happened very suddenly. Hank was a divorcé who lived here in the complex and played golf where I did. The first time I saw him at the grocery store after Jay died, he grabbed me and hugged me to express his sympathy."

Sue was a few years Hank's senior and knew his mother before she passed away. Her eventual suitor had lived with and cared for his parents until their death.

"He called right after the funeral and asked me to go out to dinner," Sue relates. "I said, 'Oh, Hank, I can't do that.' Well, we kept talking and talking and one thing led to another and I thought, 'What the heck.'"

Though Hank told Sue he'd been watching her for 20 years, it's clear he never supplanted Jay in her memory.

When asked to elaborate on her thoughts during sex, Sue

said, "With Hank, it was, 'Do I really have to go through this to be loved?' I know he loved me, because he pursued me, but I was never thrilled with sex with him."

His drinking bothered her, she finally admits. She has trouble pinning down how frequently they had sex toward the end of their marriage, when Sue was in her eighties. She eventually guesses it was five or six times a year.

"He wasn't a sexy guy," she says. "He just loved me."

ONE PARTNER, ONE LOVE

A Philadelphia native, Evelyn came to Florida in the late 1970s with her husband, Sam, a retired insurance agent.

After 66 years together, he died in 2000 and she's had "no other partners and no other desire."

Evelyn considers it *a fait accompli* that she was a virgin, but doesn't know whether she was Sam's first.

"I don't remember if I asked him," she says, "but it wouldn't have mattered if he had someone before, as long as he didn't have anyone after.

"He was the most considerate individual," she says. "He considered me as well as himself. We were very, very lucky that we found each other. We were very contented and happy together."

At 98, she has trouble providing specific answers to the survey questions.

"I don't remember [my thoughts during sex], but I know we had a wonderful sex life," she offers. Then quietly: "Once it was gone, it was gone."

Evelyn's mother died at a young age, but Evelyn learned about sex from her girlfriends, the only one in this age group to say so.

"They gave me good information."

One last question: Was her husband her only sexual partner?
"Oh, yes." As if there could be no other answer.

LIFTING THE VEIL

Thank goodness for tiny Malka and her keen memory for the intimate details of her 92 years. She stands just 4 feet, 9 inches tall—"Down from my high of 5 feet!"—and briskly welcomes me to her condo after unerringly providing complicated driving instructions.

Neat clothes and a splash of strawberry blond hair suggest a woman who's well able to care for herself. During a lengthy interview, she displays no visible health issues other than slight hearing impairment. She lives with high blood pressure and arthritis, but it's hardly a surprise when she says, "I don't tell people how old I am because they don't believe it."

For every survey question, she has spot-on answers.

What was she thinking of during sex?

"About pleasing him; I never thought of anything else. 'Is he enjoying this as much as me?'"

What was her fastest route to orgasm?

"We found that when he stimulated the clitoris, it was easiest."

When was the best sex of her life?

This was harder; no decade was any better than others from Malka's perspective. Looking back, she says even menopause didn't negatively impact her sexual desire.

But then came Reuven's diagnosis of multiple myeloma, a plasma cell cancer.

"At first, we continued having relations," she says. "As he got sicker and sicker and then took chemo . . . I found that when he was sick, I had no desire. I wasn't looking around.

"We continued having relations until about three months before he died. He was just too sick. He knew that he was not being husbandly to me, and he tried on one or two occasions. I told him, 'I have no desire now, so just don't knock yourself out.'"

But there was loving passion even at the end.

"On his deathbed he reached out and took my hand and sent a thrill through me," Malka remembers. "The next morning he was dead."

She soldiers on.

"It's 27 years now, so I've had a chance to pull my life together and go on. It hasn't been the most exciting, but it suits me."

The short-term relationship mentioned earlier, which she found unsatisfying, happened about a decade after Reuven died. But that wasn't her only attempt to reach out for companionship.

"When I started dating again, a year and a half after my husband died, all [men] wanted was sex! I'll never forget, a man took me out for dinner, a nice man, good-looking. It was a blind date. We weren't even through the salad and he said, 'Where do you want to go after this, your apartment or my apartment?'

"I said, 'I'm not going to your apartment and you're certainly not coming to mine!'"

Malka meets many people in her retirement community and not long ago invited a recently widowed man to synagogue.

"He thought that was nice, and invited me to dinner. Our third dinner, he wanted me to come up to see his apartment! I said not tonight—I made an excuse—but he kept trying to get me to come up.

"He was in his eighties, as sick as he can be, and he's looking for sex!"

Put off by his behavior, Malka mulled his possible motivations: "I don't know if it's just a desire for sex or that men have to prove their virility—you know, show that they're still capable."

Dr. Whelihan says both motivations may be true.

"It's well-known that men rate their interest in sex as primary throughout life, even when they're incapable of performing in that way. Women tell me that [their aging partner] will try for hours to penetrate them, and although the couple may engage in fondling and mutual masturbation, deep down it's the penetration the men truly long for."

For Malka, disillusioned by the suitors who followed her husband, sex went beyond simple coupling.

"Whatever happened between Reuven and I wasn't sex," she says. "It was making love and it was private.

"I waited for love and I got love," she reminisces. "He was the delight of my life."

IF I WERE TWENTY AGAIN

SOME LESSONS ARE HARDER TO LEARN THAN OTHERS.

Wouldn't it be nice if the generations of women who went before us could reach out and tell us what they learned about sex so we could avoid their mistakes? At least then our vast pool of missteps wouldn't seem so futile—and someone could learn from previous foibles.

When it comes to sex, each woman is unique, so it's especially difficult to pass along advice. What's effective for one person may very well be a deterrent to another; one woman's stimulant is another's turnoff.

Even so, it seems worthwhile to share a few insights from women whose sexuality was formed in past decades, and give younger readers a chance to learn from the experiences of those who've gone before.

So women of all ages were asked: If you knew then what you know now about your sexuality, what would you do differently if you were 20 again? Their answers were direct, wistful and poignant.

What do they have in common? Be true to yourself, choose partners carefully and learn as much as you can.

Here's what our wise women had to say:

"Even though I wouldn't give this advice to my daughter, I would

tell myself to be less inhibited. I used to be very shy and not open about sex."

—CARMEN, 46

"I wouldn't have had a baby so early. I got pregnant and married very young [17]. Basically, I would have taken things slower; I would have waited until I was old enough to know what sex was all about. I didn't have an orgasm [with a partner] till I was 24, because neither of us knew what we were doing."

—NEDIA, 73

"Be true to yourself and your needs, not just his. I wish I'd had a 52-year-old to talk to me. My mom didn't talk to me until I was in my late twenties. She told me her father had molested her, and that's when we started to talk.

I just wish someone had been honest with me about [sex]. I thought it was dirty if you weren't married, and you were bad. I felt bad about the guys I had been with and didn't enjoy it. That's part of why I became celibate. I wanted to wait till I was in love with somebody. But I think it's all a personal decision. In today's society, I don't think it's realistic to think everyone's going to wait till they're in love."

—KATRINA, 52

"I definitely would not be as inhibited as I was and not be as apprehensive about approaching women. I was pretty good at approaching men, and women wanted to approach me, but I was scared."

—CYNDI, 32

"Understand the difference between lust and love. Our need for

affection is as real as the need for sex. I would tell 20-somethings to communicate to the person what they need. So often we don't communicate what pleases us. We are all unique. There's nothing wrong with that; it's a plus. When that other person values that uniqueness, that's what will draw you together and make you one flesh."

—CANDY, 61

"I wouldn't have been taken in by the morality of the 1950s. Back then, it was a big thing to be a virgin when you married. From my perspective now, I think that's silly. I was married two months before I turned 20, and I wouldn't have married so young either. I'm not saying it was a mistake, because 54 years later we're doing fine—we've had a long and good marriage. But I do think we were too young. Things are better now with kids not rushing into marriage. My advice is to keep your sense of humor and hold hands a lot. We still do."

—ELIZABETH, 73

"Make sure you're pleased as much as your partner; don't try to please him so much. Make sure 50 percent of that pleasure is your own—I think that translates to great sex between two people."

—RENEE, 52

"I probably wouldn't have lived where I lived. I knew when I was young—maybe 4 or 5—that I was gay, and living in upstate New York was isolating. It was hard to connect with anybody; there were a lot of closed-minded folks, and trying to find like-minded people was hard. I didn't want to open up. If I was 20 again, I'd have gone to California or somewhere where [being lesbian] doesn't matter.

Also, I think I would have been quieter in general and more to myself. Regardless of what people say about times being liberal, unless you have money, [being gay] makes a difference. I'd be quieter for my own protection, because I can't do without a job. Unless you're rich, you can't promote gayism. If you need a paycheck, you can't be an advocate."

—AMY, 48

"I don't believe you can live with someone and then marry, so I wouldn't do that again. When you move in, there's a set of rules for the relationship: how it evolves, what the boundaries are. Since you aren't married, [that person] can leave anytime they want. There's no real commitment. Then suddenly you're going to marry them and it all changes. I decided after the second guy I lived with that I would not do that again."

—KYLIE, 63

"I wouldn't have been as shy as I was and as afraid of [sex] as I was. And I would have enjoyed it immediately. But I would have started at the same time [after marriage]. I don't think I would have changed that. My advice is to enjoy your mate and participate fully. And contribute to his enjoyment as well."

—RIFKI, 85

"Keep your legs closed! I wish I'd known it would hurt so much and I wish I had known how to prepare for it, like being more relaxed. I know lubricants are more common today, and it would have been great to know about them back then to help ease the pain. It was a difficult time for me, not like you read about it usually. I'm very small down there. It was never easy, and it became even more painful."

—GINA, 75

"Don't give it up. That's the same thing I've told my students and my daughter. You'll know when the time is right for you. My students used to come to school with new sneakers and no one was allowed to touch them; they even kept the price tags on. I told them, "You care more about your sneakers than you do your body." So don't give it up. Yes, it feels really good, but don't give it for just anybody.

If I had it to do all again, I would still do the same thing and be a virgin [on my honeymoon]. He's the only man I've had. For me it was the right thing."

—ROSEMARY, 60

"Get as much knowledge as you possibly can. I knew nothing."

—CATHERINE, 84

"If I was 20, I would be more cautious about the men I slept with. I'd not only ask if they had sexually transmitted diseases, but I'd ask for testing. I've had HPV [human papilloma virus] several times. I've also had genital warts. And I've learned as I've gotten older not to trust what men tell you. You should trade test results with each other. You go together to the same location, like the health department, and you go back together to pick them up.

I hope 20-somethings listen to this advice. One guy I asked about STDs said, "I should be worried about you." I was madly in love with him. I would never, never have guessed that he would put me at risk. But a lot of guys will lie to you because they don't want to use a condom."

—CHRISTINA, 55

"Before someone actually gets married, they should move in with the person and really get to know them. Because there are things

you don't realize until you're actually living with them. You'll find more bad than good. Years ago, I thought people shouldn't live together, because that's a sin according to the Catholic religion. I went out with my husband for seven years [without moving in], but after we married I found out I did not know him at all."

—BIANCA, 57

"If I was 20, I would have more sex. I missed those years because I was a virgin student; then I met my husband and didn't have sex with him [at first]. I would have liked to go out and get to know men a little more before I got engaged . . . to live a little, because then you learn a lot that way. I would use precautions like condoms not to get sick. And I would not take more than one drink, because you can lose your better judgment. If one is too much for you, don't have it. You're young; you're going to be turned on anyway. You don't need it. You have a healthy body. Besides, too much [alcohol] makes you a lousy lover. But one is good. It makes you let down the reservations."

—NINA, 59

"I would look for somebody more considerate of my sexual needs and desires, regardless of their age, race or gender."

—MARIE, 55

BRINGING UP THE REAR

WHEN WE BEGAN CRUNCHING THE NUMBERS FROM OUR 1,300 surveys to spot overarching trends, one of the first clear revelations was that many women don't like anal sex. In fact, I was told in a variety of colorful (and frank) terms, "You don't want to go there."

But the large number of women who chose this as the one thing they wish their partner would not do convinced us that a conversation was needed. When so many women— unprompted—say anal sex is their one "no-no," it indicates that a lot of men are asking to go there. Otherwise it wouldn't be surfacing as an issue.

Since an open-answered survey collects such a wide variety of answers (*every* response is a write-in), it's noteworthy when any answer garners even 10 to 15 percent of the total. The most frequently cited answer to this question, by almost 12 percent of respondents, was anal sex; even the common complaint of "rushing" was a distant second, with only 4.6 percent of the total. (When women in their nineties are dropped from the picture—which seems fair, since none evinced any knowledge of anal sex—the number moves to 13 percent.)

Anal sex is a subject that seems to polarize women: Fans and detractors are equally entrenched, though the former are harder to find. Our interviews reveal that in many cases, the survey respondents who reject anal sex have never tried it; they just know or assume they won't like it.

We'll meet the enthusiasts soon, but first, a closer look at the women who opt out of anal stimulation of any kind.

"I've never had anal sex; I'm saying 'no' sight unseen!" exclaims Addison, 46, who's been married 19 years. "It's an exit, not an entry! I tell him, 'This will never be an entry for you!'"

"I think about poop," says Hayden, who's 18. "'You're gonna get poop on your hands.' It's like poop is getting sucked back in my butt.

"My boyfriend put a finger in my butt one time and I grabbed his hand and said, 'Okay, what are you doing?' He asked if we could do anal and I said no. I don't know if it gets easier as you get older, but right now it does not interest me at all. I'm like, no way."

"Right away the pressure was too much," says 25-year-old math teacher Chelsie of the one time she tried anal sex, around age 19. "I jumped right off and said no, never again."

Now her husband of a year and a half is asking her to try.

"I joke with him and say, 'If you really want to try it, then let me stick something up you. Then if you like it, we'll give it a try.' He never goes for it. He doesn't ask often, but maybe a couple times a month to see if I'll say yes. He'll ask when I'm on my period; he'll say, 'You know, there's another kind of sex we could have.' But I don't anticipate saying yes."

"It is very painful," says Kathleen, a 28-year-old single woman. "It makes me sad that it's become kind of a 'requirement' nowadays in order to have a healthy sexual relationship."

In fact, Dr. Whelihan says many of her patients tell her that by Date 3 men are asking for anal play or anal sex. There's definitely an uptick in interest.

When asked whether she'd been approached about anal sex, Mia—the 53-year-old divorcée introduced in our kissing chapter—says, "That's every man today. It totally blows me away. In my twenties, maybe one out of a dozen guys asked for anal sex. Now everyone is asking.

"I don't know if it's a new movement . . . or maybe it's men having no respect for women. Anal sex is almost belittling, in my mind, and most women I talk to feel the same way."

"It's really not a preference for me," says Vanessa, 45, who talks about the few times her partners have attempted anal sex: "They said it was an accident or whatever, and it wasn't pleasant. I'm kind of nervous about that area, so if we're attempting doggy style, I tell him, 'Let me guide it in and go slowly,' so there are no mistakes. Because that's basically how [anal sex] happens. Guys act like it's an accident."

Vanessa is puzzled by the reactions she encounters as she tries to navigate this bedroom minefield.

"Here's what I don't understand," she explains. "They want me to have anal sex, so I say, 'Let me get something and try it on you.' And they usually say, 'Are you serious? I'm a guy; I'm not supposed to have that done.' My response is, 'When you allow me to do that to you, then we'll talk about you doing it to me.' So I turn it back around to the guy."

Despite such vehement opinions, which were expressed both in our surveys and during follow-up interviews, Dr. Mo maintains that when approached carefully and in a trusting relationship, anal sex can be an erotic addition to a couple's sex life.

"If a guy forces the issue when his girlfriend has had a few too many drinks, or tricks her by 'accidentally' initiating anal sex, it's usually fast or sudden," notes Dr. Mo, "which means the woman is going to tighten up and the pain is greater. Whatever bad impressions she harbored about the act she imagined was unpleasant, it's now *that* bad."

A slow start is the doctor's recommendation.

"Start with a finger, then move to a skinny vibrator. And use lots of lubrication!" she says.

"I will say that pressure with a finger is okay," notes Chelsie upon further questioning. "I guess [it's pleasurable] just because there are different nerve endings. But actual insertion, no."

Cheyenne, a 48-year-old bank teller, says she too has come to realize she enjoys mild anal stimulation.

"There must be some nerve there, because it makes you [climax] even faster and more intensely," she says of the times her husband uses his finger. "It's just in the last year I've allowed him to do this—no jabbing or moving around, just barely penetrating.

"If he is on top of me and tries to penetrate and it hits there, I'm like, 'No, whoa.' That quick of a moment and I think it's gonna kill me. That's how bad it hurts. I've told him, 'That one little finger, that's good!'"

Chelsie and Cheyenne are exactly right: Different nerves are being stimulated in the anal area.

A quick anatomy lesson from Dr. Mo: In the anal area, primary innervation comes from the pudendal nerve, with an assist from the inferior rectal nerve. For the clitoris, stimulation arises from several nerve groups, including the perineal, the ilioinguinal and some contribution from the same pudendal nerve (which contracts the pelvic floor).

When both areas are stimulated, expanded arousal is certainly possible.

Nevertheless, Cheyenne's enjoyment of her husband's "little

finger" embarrasses her; she hasn't even told him how much she likes it.

"I've never had anal sex and I wouldn't," she says. "It's part of the whole 'that don't belong in there; that ain't goin' in there' mindset. I can't imagine how much it would hurt, based on when he slips. I can't imagine forcing it in there."

Barbara, a 33-year-old registered nurse, has more medical knowledge than the average woman. She says after five years of marriage, she's now having the best sex of her life because her husband "knows my body."

Nevertheless, she's another respondent who vehemently proclaims: "My ass is exit only!

"My husband for years has tried to subtly hint that he wants to try [anal sex]," Barbara says, "but the tissue back there just isn't stretchy. I know physiologically it's not tissue that stretches; it's taut. He's really curious about it, but I can't bring myself to do it. I'm like, 'Let's talk about it another time.'

"I know I shouldn't knock it till I've tried," she continues, "but I just can't see how that's going to be pleasurable for me. I have this fear, honestly, that it's going to be painful. I remember when I was a teenager, I had a tilted pelvis, and every year I had a rectal exam from my gynecologist. I remember thinking, 'Good God, this is uncomfortable.'

"I know I can't equate the two; I know a trip to the gynecologist isn't sexual . . . but I can't think about it. I know gays do it, so it must stretch. Maybe I should be more open to it."

(Dr. Whelihan interjects that conducting a routine rectal exam for *any* reason on a woman under 40 is extremely atypical. "Even a tilted pelvis can be adequately evaluated through a vaginal exam," she said.)

From Barbara's uncomfortable doctor visits to Vanessa's

irritation with men who contend that their penis can't tell the difference between a vagina and a rectum, lovers who long for consensual anal sex have their work cut out for them. Some resistance and fear must often be overcome if they aspire to a sexual act their partners may have no desire for.

PAYING TO PLAY

A partner unwilling to experiment with anal sex drives some men into the arms of a girl who'll say yes to anything—for a price.

An introduction made by a friend who knew of this book's research allowed me to have a forthright conversation with Eric, a 37-year-old pimp.

I asked Eric whether the women who worked for him will allow anal sex and, if so, did it cost more?

"Out of 10 girls, three will do it 'cause they like it, one will do it for the extra money and maybe one more will do it if the dude is smooth and relaxes her," Eric says.

That leaves five who say no. Why does he think half the women won't do anal sex at all?

"Probably because guys try to slam it in . . . or they're too big. Maybe subconsciously they sense the degradation. If you don't directly talk about it with them and if they feel they're being manipulated, they feel nervous. But if you can say [what you want] directly and make them comfortable, [they'll let] you do anything you want to them."

Eric estimates that half the men who do business through him ask for anal sex —but he figures many more want it.

"The reason others won't say it is because they're nervous and scared. A lot of guys who come to me, it's about what they're not getting at home."

And the cost is higher: In the depressed economy of 2010, when a half-hour session of regular sex cost $200, Eric said the fee for a half hour of anal sex was the same as a full hour of regular sex—both were $250.

Since he had 12 years in his chosen line of work, I asked Eric why he thought men might gravitate toward anal sex.

"It's a dominating thing for a guy. You fuck a girl in the ass and you degrade her . . . you want to degrade her."

A pimp's perspective is illuminating, but obviously doesn't incorporate the viewpoint of the numerous loving couples enjoying consensual and satisfying anal sex.

So how to get there with your own spouse?

"If you're really wanting anal play," Dr. Whelihan advises men, "offer to allow anal stimulation of yourself to show that it's pleasurable and that you enjoy it as much as you think she will. Remember, it's been shown that prostate stimulation can intensify climax for men, whether it be during oral sex or vaginal penetration."

Asking your lover to arouse you this way "provides you with all the skills you need to make anal sex pleasurable for your partner. She will consciously or unconsciously show you the technique she desires, i.e., slow entry, the amount of lubrication, any other sexual stimulation for distraction and the high degree of relaxation required."

Dr. Mo warns adventuresome lovers to be aware that oftentimes, you can't easily back track.

"A lot of people find once they discover anal pleasures, that this is almost always required to finish each sexual encounter—because they can't get the same erotic arousal from the vagina," she says. "This is because the areas are innervated by two different nerve groups, which result in different sensations."

WHAT'S THE DRAW FOR MEN?

Why do we see such a large number of men who want anal sex?

Sara, a 56-year-old commercial real estate broker who's been divorced for six years, shares her thoughts:

"Maybe they think it's tighter and more resistant, or maybe it's a dominance thing. I don't know; it's probably a little bit of both. It could be an ancestral, primal thing that comes from genetics. It might go back to before we were thinking, cognitive beings—you know, kind of an animalistic thing. Think about men in jail; it's a control/dominance thing with them."

Mia, the divorcée who says she found anal sex belittling, decided to question her new boyfriend on the topic. Though they've yet to have sex, she was curious why he had already indicated interest in that variation.

"He said, 'It's because I'm so crazy about you, I want all of you.' Who knows if that's the truth? With guys they'll lie, because it's all about getting you in bed," she says.

Mia said that in her circle of maybe 35 women, only one friend admits to enjoying anal sex; the rest don't like it.

"I think it's degrading," Mia reiterates, "at least initially, when you begin dating someone. I've tried to analyze it. If you're in love with someone and you've been together awhile, it's different. It's just another avenue of sex to enjoy and explore. But when it's a new guy and you've had two or three dates, that's not to enjoy and explore; that's to exploit, in my opinion."

Jane, a 30-something registered nurse, said several of her "supposedly straight" partners have strongly desired anal sex.

"I just can't do it," she states. "More guys want it now than when I was in my twenties. Maybe it's an aggression thing, or they're angry at the world. Maybe they want some feeling of control, or to feel more superior over somebody."

Jane, who's never married, warns that "you can get tears from anal sex, and you're more at risk for STD through anal sex. For me it's mostly the pain. It's *painful*. Am I, like, just an odd woman that I don't want to allow this? Maybe I'm more normal than I think."

Plenty of women cite health concerns to explain their opposition to anal entry. Ann, a 33-year-old divorcée, said she and her boyfriend use lots of sex toys in their three or four lovemaking sessions each week.

"But I've never had anal sex," she says. "Maybe it's because of the fact that I'm constantly constipated, but it doesn't even sound interesting to me. I have serious stomach issues. It might be great, might be arousing, but I don't find it appealing. I see it as dirty, and I can't imagine enjoying that."

Dr. Whelihan understands that patients like Ann—and Grace, below—present medical issues that may either preclude anal sex or make it completely unappealing.

"With years of constipation, Ann's focus on the ass is nothing but aggravation and misery; therefore how could she think of that area as generating pleasure?"

The doctor adds, however, that for the average person, the general rule is "Any clean body part is not off-limits."

Grace, a 49-year-old librarian, first tried anal sex seven years ago, "Because it was a new relationship and it's a more popular form of sex now."

But she suffers with anal fistulas and diverticulitis, so she and her partner—they're still together—have never tried again.

"I don't have an ethic against it, but it seemed to me too painful," she clarifies, noting that her boyfriend is of above-average size. After reading more about anal sex, Grace says she decided it "doesn't seem like a natural way for this to go."

"I have a very strong belief that our culture has changed," she said. "When I grew up, having a small butt was the role model, like Twiggy. Having a large rear end wasn't important or desirable. As I've grown older, more and more there are women who are models for larger butts, like Beyoncé or Jennifer Lopez. It's much more prevalent. More marketing and appreciation of the butt has naturally led to more objectifying that as an ideal for women—and it creates an obsession in men."

Grace, who's white with a black boyfriend, said she believes the idealization of women for the size of their butts is much more prevalent in black culture.

When asked whether she thinks this preoccupation with "junk in the trunk" and curvy butts has a direct correlation on men asking their partners for anal sex, Grace says, "Absolutely."

She also credits easy access to Internet porn with creating curiosity in men.

"From what my boyfriend and some of the men he knows say, the best porn movies are the ones that contain anal sex."

Nonetheless, after their initial foray, her partner has never put pressure on her for anal sex.

Daphne, a single woman of 28, moved to America from Poland seven years ago, and blames porn for the unfavorable opinion she has formed of American men's sexual preferences.

"Things are much more exposed here than in Poland . . . men watch lots of porn, and whatever they see they want to do. It doesn't matter if it's pleasurable to you. I always say I'm not going to do [anal sex]. I use that hole for one purpose and that's it. It's disgusting to think people wouldn't mind."

Daphne believes men sometimes request anal sex so they won't have to use protection against pregnancy.

"You might hear you won't get STDs that way," she says, "but men try different tricks. I know that you can. But some women aren't educated and might go for that.

"What really disgusts me is when men complain about tightness of women after they have children," she concludes. "They say they want the tightness of the anus and that's why they enjoy it. Some women are insecure and they'll do it. They think, 'If I don't give it to my husband, he will go elsewhere and he will get it.'"

Which is pretty much what happened to another woman I spoke with. Gabriella was 48 and toward the end of her 13-year marriage when her soon-to-be ex husband wanted to have anal sex.

"I said absolutely not; I told him I'm not an object," says the pretty high school teacher. "He told me I was not tight anymore, so he wanted it tight again. Right now I'm laughing [as she relates her story], but it made me cry for a long time. I tell him I have three kids; I cannot be as tight as the first time. I thought it was mean, disrespectful and nasty to say it."

Such men naturally give women a repugnance for anal sex, but under all kinds of circumstances, other women freely choose to travel this path.

"It's all about how it's delivered," says Dr. Whelihan. "Is he trying to sneak in or is he saying, 'I love you so much I want to penetrate all of you.' It can't be just a self-serving thing for him. So often the woman is left to feel, 'Well, good for you, but not so good for me.' It has to be more than just, 'Your vagina is baggy and I need a tighter squeeze.'"

THE OTHER SIDE

Once she leaves the office, Dr. Whelihan makes it a point to research the male opinion on matters of sexual desire. During medical lectures, at business meetings and cocktail parties, even on airplanes, she zealously solicits the male point of view.

As a result, she has some clues about why anal sex appeals to men.

"I think they want it because it's naughty and they see it in porn, which is now simple to access online and represents a *huge* change in our culture, one which surely contributes to the popularity of anal sex.

"Plus, it's something they haven't done—they're just curious or being frisky. You have to remember that men's lives revolve around their ability to penetrate.

"Another reason they want it is that it's rumored—rightly so—to be a tighter opening and therefore they want to experience 'the grab.'"

Why are men in their sixties and seventies getting on the bandwagon?

Dr. Mo says men with psychological aspects of erectile dysfunction need something intensely erotic to get them excited. "That's why they're asking for it," she explains.

It's possible, she continues, that a small percent of men—maybe 10 percent—are pressuring their female partners for anal sex because they have a predisposition for bisexuality or homosexuality.

"For this minority, anal sex carries even greater appeal," she says. "It could be we're discovering the percentage of the population who are homosexual, but practicing heterosexuals."

Elizabeth, a 39-year-old divorcée who said she had anal sex just twice with her husband of 13 years, is now dating a 33-year-old man. In their two years together, they have added anal sex to the mix a handful of times.

"It's okay every now and then, if he wants to try it once in a blue moon, but it's not something I'd want to do as a regular part of our lovemaking," Elizabeth said, adding that they use plenty of lubricant. "He may want to try it when we've been drinking, but he'll check on me and say, 'Is it okay?' He'll do it doggy style, but then go in the other way."

Dr. Mo says forewarned is forearmed.

The anal canal is a very tight, circular, muscular band that doesn't have the same stretch and elasticity as the vagina.

"The concerns are that rapid or excessive stretching can cause tearing," she says. "Tearing of external skin around the anal opening, called a fissure, is not such a big deal. It's painful but not harmful, and heals quickly, usually within 48 hours. But tearing of the fascia or muscle fibers can lead to permanent trauma, resulting in reduced sphincter tone or tightness of the sphincter. A consequence of this could be a relaxation in that area or even fecal incontinence."

This danger is part of why prostitutes charge extra for anal sex.

A higher rate of STD infection also accompanies anal sex: There is more trauma involved, and traumatized tissue makes for an easier entry point for diseases such as HIV or gonorrhea.

FANS OF THE FANNY

Among women, the practice does have its zealous fans.

"To me, I like it because it's the ultimate orgasm," says Lakia, 44. "I feel it everywhere, like an explosion on the Fourth of July. Once you have it, you want to lie down. I have a smile on my face . . . I need two cigarettes and a nap!

"I've had vaginal orgasms that were over-the-top too," she continues, "but an anal orgasm is like lobster instead of crab. It is just awesome."

Lakia responds so well to anal sex that it is sometimes her go-to position.

"I've been with some guys who didn't really hit my G-spot or give me an orgasm, so we'd try [anal sex] and it would give me an orgasm."

She notes that her G-spot is very sensitive, as opposed to her clitoris, which is less so.

"Some guys give me oral clitoral stimulation, but that doesn't really do it for me," she says. "Everybody's different, of course, but when my girlfriends say, 'Oh, I'm scared it'll hurt, I don't want to try it,' not to gross you out, but I say, 'You have bowel movements bigger than a man's penis.' And they say, 'But it's coming out.'

"To each his own," she summarizes. "I know what I like."

Lakia, who became sexually active at age 15 and has been with perhaps 50 partners, first tried anal sex in her twenties at her lover's request because she was on her cycle.

"It wasn't the most pleasant thing because that was my first time," she recounts. "Once I got used to it, I liked it a little more. I like to try new things, because I get bored with the regular missionary positions or the man always wanting the woman to be on top. I like new and exciting things."

With larger partners, Lakia says anal penetration can be difficult, "But if you're on top, you control how much goes in . . . they just have to slow down. If he's behind you [he might] want to go too fast, too deep. They rush because they're so excited about being back there, since it's tight. It's like being with a virgin."

Lakia and her fiancé have only tried anal sex a few times, she says, so it's still painful "because I don't do it regularly."

There are other things she adamantly refuses to consider.

"I've seen porn videos where people go from anus to vagina. That is disgusting. I'm not doing that . . . it's crazy and it's not clean. After anal sex, if you change the condom, shower, whatever . . . *then* sometimes I want to have vaginal sex."

Lakia doesn't know why men want this: "Maybe the excitement of having two holes to be in almost at the same time," she speculates.

(Notes Dr. Whelihan: "I always remind patients that you can go from front to back but *not* back to front without washing first. Or a couple may choose to use a condom in back and then take it off for vaginal sex.")

"One thing about anal sex, you *have* to be in the mood for it," cautions Lakia. "You have to be relaxed. If you're too timid or nervous, it's not going to work, because you're going to lock up."

One last tip, and it's a graphic one: "Your diet has to be good. You have to drink a lot of water and eat vegetables; it kind of loosens you up back there. If you're regular it's a little bit more comfortable. And make sure you're lubricated. That's important, although sometimes I don't have to be lubricated if I'm really turned on."

Of course, Lakia isn't alone in her enthusiasm for anal sex. Macy, a 34-year-old divorcée, shares her experience.

"With anal sex, a lot of people are turned off first of all because it can be messy, and it hurts if you don't relax your body," says the X-ray technician. "With anything such as having a catheter or giving blood or getting an IV, you have to relax. That's true with anything going into your body that isn't normal.

"I have to say the first time I tried it was definitely a little painful, but it was something I wanted to try again—because at the same time there was pleasure."

Years before she had anal sex, Macy shares that a lover had

used his tongue to explore her anal region. "I was like, wow. It felt really, really good. I realized [anal sex] was something I'd want to try one day."

That day came when she was in her late twenties, but the experience made her realize she needed to be more secure with her partner.

"It was a long-distance relationship and we didn't have the comfort level we needed. The second guy I had anal sex with is the guy I really liked it with, and we continue to have sex—and anal sex—every now and then, though we're not in a relationship."

With this particular lover, who's nine years younger, Macy says she orgasms most easily during anal sex with one of them rubbing her clitoris.

"That's a change for me," she shares. "I used to reach orgasm faster when I was on top, but maybe three years ago I began to change. Now when I'm on top, it gets me closer, but I don't feel like I'm going to orgasm. But I can tell you it's almost instantaneous when he gets behind me."

Linda, who's 46 and works in the accounting field, says her husband of 23 years sometimes wants to have anal sex.

"How do you know if you don't like something if you don't try it?" she asks. "Once we were on a cruise and we tried it. It wasn't easy, but I tried. Other times he touched me around there and I found it to be totally exciting. If he goes in just enough to get past the barrier, just the tip of his penis, it makes me come. If he teases and it doesn't hurt, I like it.

"It's not something I want all the time, but every once in a while. My preference is when we combine [vaginal] penetration with a vibrator [which she uses] and anal stimulation."

Louise, 27, tried anal sex with her lover when they began

dating seven years ago, but it was uncomfortable, so she just told him to stop.

Then last year, in an early-morning scenario when they were sleepily having sex in the spoon position, she realized her relaxed state had made anal sex possible. Even her boyfriend was surprised. "It did feel like he was in the vaginal area and then I dozed off for a second. When I woke up, I just had this rush inside my whole body. I was like, 'Holy shit, we're having anal sex.'"

The couple tried it again that same night, and Louise estimates that they now have anal sex about 15 percent of the time. She and her lover, who she says is average size, don't use lubrication, and she doesn't require simultaneous clitoral stimulation in order to orgasm.

"You have to relax, drown out everything else," she says. "Think of the ocean. It's a different type of stimulation. It's totally different than vaginal sex. You get this rush; I get goose bumps and chills. I have harder orgasms . . . and quicker."

Clearly not everyone is going to become a fan of anal sex, but it's worthwhile to examine the emotional and physical ramifications of exploring this variation. Keep an open mind and a relaxed body and you may be surprised. Don't take the health consequences lightly, but if you follow some general rules of safety, anal play can add a new erotic edge to your lovemaking.

CHEAT SHEET FOR GUYS

AT COCKTAIL PARTIES, BARS AND HAPPY HOURS—ANYWHERE people are feeling flirty and open—Dr. Whelihan often finds herself surrounded by men hanging on her every word. She's plenty charismatic, but not a supermodel, so why the crowd?

It's the novelty factor: After all the mystery and confusion, men are stunned and delighted to discover a bona fide expert who's willing to pass on straightforward information about what women really want in the bedroom. Dr. Mo's neutral manner fascinates them; she addresses sex without sensationalism, as if it's on a par with high blood pressure or weight control. The men press close, and some linger as the crowd thins, hoping to capitalize on their unexpected encounter by scoring a private moment to share their story—and hopefully receive a bit of Dr. Mo's insight or advice to apply to their lives.

What we're offering here, gentlemen, is a seat at the table during happy hour, as Dr. Whelihan presents a summary of *Kiss and Tell's* best lessons and elaborates on eight things men must understand about women's desire.

"Guys *want* to be good at this," she says. "They are eager for information. Men are my best students, because they are willing to do any of the homework assignments in hopes that it means more sex!"

So pay attention, men. These crib notes are the abridged version of what we learned from 1,300 women about sexual desire. Absorb these few lessons, and you may just unlock your woman's deepest reserves of passion.

1) First, a little science: You should know that the steroid hormone known as testosterone is such a huge factor in your life that it most likely motivated you to seek lovemaking tips in this book. The concentration levels of testosterone in men are roughly eight times higher than those in the majority of women on the planet. Do *not* underestimate this difference. Granted, women routinely fail to grasp the enormous effect testosterone has on your gender and how it affects your sex drive, but men are equally ignorant of what the lack of testosterone means for women. Without that hormone coursing through their veins and urging them toward sex, women must rely on other (external) enticements.

It's not that a mother of three doesn't love her husband; it's that without the incessant biological push her partner gets from testosterone, she's forced to wait on other physical or emotional stimuli to rise above the clamor and pull her toward a sexual encounter. This is *your* call to action.

This need for other stimuli is why Dr. Mo tells women not to turn down their partners' requests for sex: "Instead say, 'I don't know; try to convince me,'" she advises. "That way, guys are called upon to do a little seduction, to remind their partner of how stimulating foreplay and sex can be." A woman's sex drive is set on neutral, says Dr. Mo. "A smart man knows how to coax her out of neutral and propel her forward."

2) Beware of courting behavior and the false expectations it encourages. Yes, yes, we know you have thoughts of sex every 52 seconds on average and that your fantasies are for an endless

stream of willing sex partners. But let's agree that most men's reality is a tad tamer—and when it comes to doing the deed, there is a broad range for what's normal.

Know this: People with an average sex drive pair up once a week; those with a high drive have sex once a day and those with a low drive have sex once a month. All of these libidos are *normal.*

Problems arise when partners from opposite ends of the spectrum find themselves paired. This happens because during courting behavior—as women are often wooed with flowers, dinners and compliments—their libidos are stimulated by the attention, causing them to desire sex more frequently than usual.

When that wooing behavior ceases, and everyday routines set in, a woman's libido may fall back to her norm, whatever that is.

"This is why you need to know your level of interest and convey it to your partner early on," says Dr. Whelihan. "New relationships cause tremendous surges of dopamine in the brain, which propel us toward sex. But over time, this effect is blunted. We return to a normal state, and those surges only occur through purposeful seduction, which may include reading erotica or watching a sexy flick. It takes work and continual effort."

Since the range of "normal" for frequency of sex goes from daily to monthly, tying your self-worth to the number of times your partner has sex with you makes little sense. Guys shouldn't make the mistake of thinking that if a woman loves them, she'll always want to have sex. That's simply not so.

3) Don't move in long-term. (In other words, don't get too comfy in her vagina.) Some men have taken women's "you finish too fast in bed" complaint to mean that extended penetration time is desired. Not true. Most women—especially married

women—prefer shorter periods of penetration.

"Now, don't get me wrong," says Dr. Whelihan. "They *love* foreplay, especially clitoral stimulation, because that leads to orgasm. Once she reaches orgasm, penetration is welcome, but generally requested for 10 or 15 minutes only. Busy women commonly complain that 25 minutes is just too long and they would rather not get started at all than to put up with that."

Soreness and damage to vaginal tissue also are possible during extended penetration.

Read the expression on your mate's face: If she looks like she is picking out wallpaper in her head or creating a grocery list, it is time to wrap it up.

4) Your most-ignored sex organ is your ears. Use them to *listen* to what your lover wants in bed. Our survey proves that every woman has a unique sexual profile, so don't assume what worked with one partner is right for another. Quick example: "Dirty talk" was frequently mentioned by our survey takers as a turn-on . . . and just as frequently listed as the one thing they wish their partner would not do. Avoid a huge blunder here by discovering your partner's preference *before* sex.

If you're in an exclusive relationship, you should already know that the same routine month after month will dull even the most sensuous connection. Therefore, ask your lover gentle questions about likes and dislikes.

That does *not* mean you should unleash a litany of queries in bed. A good number of our survey takers criticized bedroom chatter, often because women are concentrating on a fantasy in order to achieve orgasm. So to them, open-ended questions such as "What do you want next?" or, "Do you want something different?" are a distracting turnoff. Better questions are the occasional, "Do you like this slower or faster?" or, "How about trying this?"

And don't be afraid to use those neglected sex organs outside the bedroom as well. Over a glass of wine at dinner, ask whether there's something special she'd like to try, or tell her an idea you have. Women carry vestiges of a myth that the "right" partner will automatically understand her body and answer its every desire on every occasion, but that belief is unreal. Help her let go of it by educating yourself on what she likes and growing into that perfect lover.

5) Don't be an ass. So you're feeling experimental and would love to try anal sex, but your partner hasn't shown herself to be willing to accommodate back-door traffic. Be aware: Popular pornography has greatly exaggerated the enthusiasm females have for this variation. Nevertheless, you have a much better chance of success if you follow a few guidelines.

First, never "accidentally" attempt anal sex. Without preparation, your partner will not be sufficiently relaxed, so never force anything. Start small—think a finger—and use lubrication. If she tenses up, back off and *slow down.*

Second, remember that most women who say they enjoy anal sex also require simultaneous clitoral stimulation. Act accordingly.

Last, if you're convinced you can make anal play exciting for her, show her you're serious by allowing anal stimulation of yourself. It will help you become familiar with the sensations you're hoping she'll enjoy and the high degree of relaxation required for this variation to succeed.

6) Be flexible on your timing. Don't assume the bedtime sex you crave is your partner's choice as well. Yes, it helps you unwind, relax and fall asleep—but women tend to be exhausted at this time of night. Sex can feel like one more thing they have to do. *Ask your mate* what time of day she prefers sex. You may

hear "late morning" or "before dinner in the late afternoon." Use this information! By always delaying sex until bedtime, you increase the chances of encountering a fatigued partner with little enthusiasm for sex and the perceived energy it requires.

7) Kiss her! Once upon a time, you used your kisses to let a woman know of your desire. Remember that? Compare those early kisses—with all their passion and pent-up yearning—to the ones you now offer as a prelude to sex. Do they measure up? If so, congratulations. You're probably having some great sex. If not, vow to spend two minutes a day passionately kissing your mate. The results will amaze you. That's because kissing is the most frequently mentioned answer to the question of what stimulates desire—for women of all ages.

8) Show appreciation. You knew this was coming . . . the directive to compliment your partner. Unless they're comfortable with their softer side, men find this activity difficult. But it works, so listen up.

Recognize and acknowledge the importance of your wife's role as a mother or as keeper of the house or as partner extraordinaire. Acknowledge to her how hard she works and how special she is to you. Often just a little help with the housework or watching the kids so she can slip away to the gym or out for a cocktail with friends lets her know you're in her corner.

And how does a woman feel about a man in her corner?

You're the one with the testosterone. We think you can figure that one out!

LESSONS LEARNED

THE TWO YEARS I SPENT CONDUCTING INTERVIEWS FOR *Kiss and Tell* were the most educational ones of my life. My very first interview took place in the home of Dulce, the "yes-we-really-have-sex-every-day" woman who's featured in the "Kiss Me You Fool" chapter.

I sat at her modest dining room table while she unspooled the remarkable details of the romance she'd shared with her husband of 32 years, wondering whether it was okay to stare as she pointed to pieces of furniture and places in the room where they'd had sex. I was thrilled by her unvarnished candor and secretly hoped Freddy would come home from work in time for me to get a glimpse of the mythic man whose kisses and lovemaking had kept his wife purring for decades.

I didn't meet Freddy, but as I left their house, I knew Dulce's sex life would be one of the most joyful, active histories I was going to collect for the entire book—and I was right. She proved to be a fabulous introduction to the private world of women's desire that I was entering.

Even though Dulce set the bar high for my expectations, the women of *Kiss and Tell* never let me down. Along the way, representatives from every decade surprised and delighted me. Their individual stories were riveting—every single one. No one was tedious; no one described an uninteresting life.

My hope is that, like me, you fell in love with these women as they open-heartedly shared their most personal experiences and innermost thoughts—often for the first time.

I laughed out loud with Rifki as the 85-year-old described an unforeseen challenge of senior sex: Her skinny boyfriend's sharp hip bones and elbows poke her when he climbs on top! I sat transfixed on the tiny porch of her seniors' community apartment as this charming woman explained how Elias, her husband of 55 years, had calmed her fears of sex on their honeymoon, been a patient lover, introduced her to oral sex and always made sure she had orgasms first. Though her sex life began with misgivings, Rifki happily exclaimed, "Once we started—oh boy!"

I cheered when Catherine told me of her first orgasm, at age 82, and teared up when she sweetly assured me she never felt resentment for a life path that hadn't led to intimate satisfaction sooner.

I tried to keep my jaw from dropping to the floor as Jackie, a very attractive 67-year-old, talked about having sex with her first husband three times a day . . . for two decades! Actually it was for 20 years, 4 months and 20 days, and I'm sure if I'd been in a similar marriage, I could pinpoint its length with Jackie's accuracy. No other woman described a partner this demanding.

As the interviews unfolded, my misconceptions and judgments fell away, one by one. I loved how empowered the teens were, how luminous the twenties. I was thrilled at the richness of women in mid-life, and struggled to give their full lives expression within a single chapter. They had much to say, and I wanted to provide a worthy platform. I was reassured to see that life could still be messy and real for women in their seventies and

I was overcome with tenderness for the ladies in their eighties. Each woman made an impression on my heart; after every interview I felt buoyant, but also humbled and grateful for their candor and generosity of spirit, not to mention the trust they invested in me by holding nothing back.

Whenever I was caught off guard by a surprising revelation, I was deeply thankful for the new material, because it meant I'd be able to share the unusual tidbit in *Kiss and Tell*, where other women, even if only a few, could read it and identify with the experience.

In this way, the women of *Kiss and Tell* hold up the mirror for all of us. I had the privilege of looking in that mirror first. In these women's stories, I recognized pieces of my own sexuality, my own insecurities, my own preferences. No two women are identical, of course, but we share enough common ground that early on in the process, I came to feel completely comfortable in the big sea of sexuality where we all swim.

This sea is where Dr. Whelihan already lives. Because of her immersion in the lives of her patients, she already knew what I came to understand: We are all the same.

Every one of us, no matter our age, is trying to find our way in and out of this crazy piece of the human essence that is our sexuality. And we are trying to stay on the path of discovery, but it's confusing, and so occasionally we question whether we've wandered afield. Sometimes we're nervous about exploring; sometimes we're confident. And though we glance at the routes other women are taking, we're hesitant to show our insecurity by asking directions because we're pretty sure everyone else has discovered a more direct route to intimate satisfaction than we have.

We're afraid we're different, even abnormal.

Not true. The women of *Kiss and Tell* demonstrate we're all normal. We are smart, complex, loving, adventurous, insecure, searching, shy, funny, sincere, reticent and empowered beings. And far from being a weakness, these complexities are our strengths.

The differences I discovered among the women of *Kiss and Tell* often arose from the era in which they were born or the cultural pressures at the time. Naturally, how they were raised played a part, as did their reactions to the circumstances of life, including the challenges of abuse, alcoholism, illness and affairs. Their experiences are true reflections of the trials we all face in life.

The goal for each of us—from the 15-year-old virgin to the 80-year-old who yearns for companionship—is to balance our ability to take leaps of faith with our inner sense of what we want.

Along the way, keep in mind that no one is smarter about you and your body than you.

If you're struggling to decide whether to have sex for the first time, know that if the reasons aren't right *for you*, you may come to regret the choice. If you're an exhausted mom in your forties with a full-time job and no energy for sex, know that this isn't the end of your sexual story, that empty nests often bring a blossoming of sexual energy. If you're feeling dry and despondent after menopause, find a doctor and discuss hormone therapy; there's ample evidence that it can enhance your libido. If you're 80 and discover that you have surprising feelings for the gentleman down the hall in the seniors' home, ask your granddaughter to bring you some condoms, make sure the lock on your door works and go for it with joy.

These are the things Dr. Whelihan tells her patients every

day, and so this book becomes the wider conversation she has wanted to have with all women.

"Every day I see women who are dissatisfied with their sex lives, and most take responsibility by reporting they have no desire," she states. "But I am here to tell you, women don't have low desire for sex, they have low desire for the sex they're having. At the end of the day, my patients truly love sex. Most of them are even orgasmic on a regular basis.

"But they need permission to enjoy sex. My mission is to 'normalize' the thoughts, behaviors and desires of women and give them a green light to enjoy sexual intimacy. I want them to learn to turn off negative thoughts during sex and sink into a sensual awareness of their bodies, to simply embrace what feels good.

"And I want them to relay this information to their partner as best they can, because I'm convinced that most men will do anything to please their lover at that moment."

So there it is—your homework assignment, or perhaps your marching orders. And maybe just the keys to the kingdom . . .

Because it's not just that sex matters, it's that in sex, *you* matter. Your desires, your preferences and your fantasies continue to matter throughout every stage of your life. So don't sell yourself short.

While I worked on this book, friends couldn't resist the occasional query about how my increasing knowledge was affecting my own sex life. Typical of my generation, I consider bedroom confessions mostly private, so without the anonymity afforded the women in this book, I'm not tempted to kiss and tell.

Still, if we should ever meet and I learn you've read this book, and you learn I'm the writer, I predict we'll feel an immediate kinship due to the cozy chats about sex we've shared here. And I'm pretty sure we'll recognize the sparkle in each other's eyes.

SURVEY QUICKIES

WHAT IS YOUR QUICKEST ROUTE TO ORGASM?

It's not so quick anymore. 75, WIDOWED

Oral clitoral stimulation. Duh. 36, DIVORCED

All routes are closed. 73, widowed

There is no quick route; it usually takes about 45 minutes or I don't have an orgasm at all. 45, DIVORCED

Never had one. 33, DIVORCED

On top, with no penetration. 48, SINGLE

Masturbation in shower. 46, MARRIED

Nipple stimulation while having sex at the same time. 30, SINGLE

Feet over his head, with him on top. 22, SINGLE

I'm not sure if I've ever had an orgasm. Everyone tells me I would know! 34, SINGLE

Recently, it's oral sex with finger in anus, but nothing bigger. And don't tell my husband it actually is a turn-on. Something about it doesn't seem right to me and it's embarrassing that it actually turns me on. 48, MARRIED

Six batteries and a beautiful woman (my partner). 46, LESBIAN

WHAT STIMULATES YOUR DESIRE?

Wearing tight thong underwear. 61, DIVORCED

Anticipation. 29, SINGLE AND 59, DIVORCED

Sexy books. 86, MARRIED

Right now, nothing. 75, MARRIED

At my age, anything! 66, MARRIED

Being treated like the most special woman in the world and being told how much I am appreciated. 28, SINGLE

When my husband does things around the house and I feel appreciated. 57, MARRIED

Long, passionate kissing, which I hear stops after marriage. 56, SINGLE

His passion for me. 70, WIDOWED

Him dancing and stripping for me; me dancing and stripping for him. 52, MARRIED

Controlling the emotions, actions of my partner. 36, married

Discussing the act beforehand, kind of like verbal foreplay. 33, SINGLE

Touching my breasts, feeling desired, smacking my behind, talking dirty. 79, WIDOWED

Watching porn. 49, MARRIED

A man I can't have! 36, MARRIED

Being thin. 63, MARRIED

The smell of suntan lotion or sunscreen. It takes me back to my youth at the beach. 50, MARRIED

Anything, since I'm not getting any. 66, SINGLE

My opinion: The bigger the dick, the less he thinks he has to do. It's all about them. The smaller the dick, usually the sweeter, more compassionate the guy is and goes out of his way to please. Bigger isn't always better! 45, DIVORCED

WHAT IS THE ONE THING YOU WISH YOUR PARTNER WOULD NOT DO IN REGARDS TO SEX?

Think that stating "Let's do it!" is foreplay. 46, MARRIED

Watch TV during. 47, LESBIAN

Rush to stimulate my clitoris. 54, DIVORCED

Take too long to finish on purpose. When my husband does that, I'm usually sore and annoyed. 37, MARRIED

Too much foreplay can ruin it for me. 28, SINGLE

Put finger inside; it reminds me of my ob/gyn. 26, MARRIED

Smoke afterward. 80, WIDOWED

Leave his socks on! 28, SINGLE

Take a Viagra and not tell me. 71, MARRIED

Ask questions about his performance. 35, MARRIED

Blow on my personal spot. 47, MARRIED

Lose his erection. 67, MARRIED

Ask me to shave my pubic hair. It is irritating for me during

sex. 26, MARRIED

Ask "So, are we having sex today?" 26, SINGLE

Turn the lights on! 62, DIVORCED

Stop and text her mother back. 19, LESBIAN

I have never been comfortable with oral sex. 45, MARRIED

Work so hard in trying to give me an orgasm. 65, DIVORCED

Look at me while doing oral, trying to look in my eyes. Ugh! 47, MARRIED

Drool during kissing. 41, MARRIED

Try to get in butt! 67, MARRIED

Go for time four, five or six. I'm worn out and on fire by that time! OMG! But I'm not complaining at my age. 46, DIVORCED

Just start right out by grabbing my crotch. 49, MARRIED

Make me swallow during oral. 66, DIVORCED

Use a toy without his human touch. 45, DIVORCED

Make me feel guilty when I don't want it. 39, MARRIED

Say "Am I hurting you?" especially when he is very small. 61, DIVORCED

Don't 'motorboat' my vagina during oral. It's stupid and ridiculous and I'm not a porn star. 23, SINGLE

Have intercourse without any part of his body touching mine—like I was a hole in the wall. 62, DIVORCED

I do not like spanking or slapping. 58, WIDOWED

Talk. 43, MARRIED

Think I only want his penis stuck in my vagina. What a turn-off. 60, SINGLE

Try to pleasure me with no knowledge of the anatomy. It becomes so frustrating; it's a turnoff. 76, MARRIED

Say "fuck, yeah" and grunt possessively. 35, MARRIED

Use toys for a long time. I lose sensitivity down there. 57, MARRIED

Ask me to lick his toes. 49, MARRIED

Bug me about having anal sex, which isn't something I'm into. I wish men would just be satisfied with two holes! 53, DIVORCED

Stop asking me if I am coming just because I moan. 39, MARRIED

The same thing over and over again! 64, MARRIED

Fumble around with breasts. I don't think they know what to do with them! 49, DIVORCED

Think and act like a guy. Sometimes my partner does and it is a turn-off. 46, LESBIAN

He sometimes spits to lubricate. Yuck. 31, SINGLE

Wake me at 5:15 a.m. for sex. 75, SINGLE

Come to bed with an unshaven face and unbrushed teeth. 39, MARRIED

Attempt to re-stimulate me after an orgasm. 71, MARRIED

Remind me that he's taken Viagra and give me a time frame. 73, MARRIED

I'm used to it after 37 years, but at first I didn't like him to

immediately get up and wash up. 58, MARRIED

Kiss me after oral sex. 49, married

Finish before me, but as we get older it happens more frequently. 28, MARRIED

Ask questions during sex. 56, MARRIED

WHAT'S IN YOUR BRAIN DURING SEX? (WHAT ARE YOU THINKING ABOUT?)

Sometimes I think of homework. 26, SINGLE

The image of an erect penis. 46, MARRIED

Fantasy sex. 46, MARRIED

Songs. I sing certain songs in my mind. "Roll me over, in the clover. Do it again, do it again." 67, MARRIED

Hurry up. 81, MARRIED

Am I doing this right? 21, SINGLE

How wonderful this could be. 77, MARRIED

I could be doing something more productive. 26, SINGLE

I want to have an orgasm. 71, MARRIED

Why does oral give me an orgasm and not his penis? 28, MARRIED

How fat I am. 34, MARRIED

I sure don't want to be pregnant! 93, WIDOW

George Clooney. 47, MARRIED

I think about climaxing if it's good. If it's bad, I think of things

I need to get done. 31, DIVORCED

I wonder what I need to do for him to finish. 27, SINGLE

Just before I orgasm, I sometimes imagine that I am a man. 50, SINGLE

Relaxation ... it took years to get my dad's anger over his daughter being sexually active out of my head. 40, MARRIED

I'm not married. I shouldn't be doing this, but I can't help it! 42, SINGLE

I hope my partner is not thinking about someone else. 28, single

Faster ... slower ... up ... down. 53, MARRIED

I'm thinking about other muscular, hot, sexy men; orgies; sex with other people watching; or even having sex with other men while my husband watches. 44, MARRIED

Things I can do that will make him nuts. 57, MARRIED

Depends. Sometimes it's "I hope he's enjoying this." Sometimes it's "I hope this is over soon." 34, MARRIED

Fantasies of things I would never do. 62, MARRIED

Please don't touch my fat belly! 43, MARRIED

Let it be good this time. 68, MARRIED

Not to be hurt (because I'm) too dry. 83, MARRIED

Making sure he doesn't come before I do. 46, MARRIED

How nice it is to be this close — how inferior it is compared to when we were young. 55, MARRIED

If I'm making him as happy as he seems. 18, SINGLE

Where are the old feelings? 58, MARRIED

Should I tell him what he should do to make me feel good or should I let him find out on his own? 29, SINGLE

Being younger! 50, MARRIED

Chores I have to do, which drives my husband insane. 51, MARRIED

What can I do for him to understand this is or is not what I want. 47, SINGLE

Lately, "Are you done yet?" 49, MARRIED

Reaching a climax together. 72, MARRIED

Get it over with. 73, MARRIED

I usually have fantasies about being spanked or held down. Sometimes it's more than one partner. It seems to always involve being dominated, although in real life, that's never happened. 37, MARRIED

Sex, Sex, Sex — Who can think of anything else! 86, WIDOW

Am I really enjoying this? I should be cleaning, washing clothes, etc. 75, MARRIED

God, I wish he'd lose weight. 71, MARRIED

If I will know when I'm climaxing. 20, MARRIED

I'm hoping I can get to orgasm. 87, WIDOWED

Usually what I need to get done during the week. 45, DIVORCED

I wonder why it's not as good as it used to be. 69, MARRIED

Why am I here? 75, WIDOWED

DESCRIBE THE BEST SEX OF YOUR
LIFE, HOW OLD AND WHY ...

In my 40s, with my husband, in a car at a concert venue while waiting to pick up our teenage son from a concert. Excitement and danger! 69, MARRIED

Probably in my forties. Now it's quality, not quantity. He really tries hard to please me; makes sure I have an orgasm. When we were first together, I was fearful of talking about orgasms and how I have them. No secrets anymore. 44, MARRIED

Fifty-plus; stayed in bed all day. No food, no TV, no music, just sex. 60, MARRIED

I was 22 years old, at home with my husband (then fiancé), in my old room. The fact that my family was in the house made it adventurous. It was the first time I squirted and I didn't care who heard me; it felt incredible! 23, MARRIED

In my forties. I discovered how to give myself an orgasm, since a man hadn't been able to. 56, MARRIED

I was 30; it was with the first guy after my divorce, who was the second sexual partner of my life. It was the first time I had an orgasm during intercourse. 52, MARRIED

Age 28 in Nova Scotia on a cliff. The air smelled of cool pine, the whole day was foreplay, no distractions, just bliss. 63, MARRIED.

I was 41; had a huge mental connection to my partner. 48, MARRIED

It was with my husband when we were in college and not married. He rented a room from an old lady and we had to be extremely quiet so she thought we were studying. It was the thrill of getting away with it. 45, MARRIED

Outdoors at the beach. I was 18. 45, MARRIED

I was 50 and had a massage with a cute, buff, 35-year-old massage therapist. Talk led to touching and sex. He had great technique. It was so great to know that an overweight, 50-year-old could still turn on a young guy. He made me feel desirable and sexy and I needed that! 52, MARRIED

The older I get, the better it seems to get. 41, MARRIED

I was in my 40s; just beginning a new relationship. I had three people together. 67, MARRIED

At 26, in a car parked where we shouldn't be. 65, MARRIED

In my forties, after my divorce. It was the first time in my life it was all about me and when I get mine first. 45, DIVORCED

In the back seat of a limo on our 25th anniversary. 64, MARRIED

I think I'm starting to enjoy it more now at 35. 35, MARRIED

Everything now; no more inhibitions. 81, MARRIED

I was 25 years old. It was after a lengthy roll-playing session involving picking up my lover as a hitchhiker. 50, SINGLE

Not sure I've found that yet. 45, DIVORCED

I was in my early 30s and it was with a female. I think it was so great because it was so forbidden. It was all consuming — mentally, physically, emotionally. I'd never felt anything like it before and have never felt anything like it since. 38, MARRIED

When I was pregnant. I didn't have to worry about getting pregnant. That was freedom! 48, MARRIED

The best sex I ever had in my life was at the age of 32. He was from Jamaica and his penis was so big that when we had sex

it filled my whole vagina. He hit every single spot and slowly made love to me. I came so hard I shivered. 33, SINGLE

I was 20; he was my second partner. I had previously not enjoyed sex because the first was quite large. I was physically compatible with the second and was very attracted to him. 29, MARRIED

It was around age 30, with my discovery of the vibrator. 54, SINGLE

It just keeps getting better and better as I learn to relax and trust myself. 74, MARRIED

The best sex was a period of frequent, hours-long foreplay and stop and start and finish together. We were in our early 30s and this was our decade of delight. 62, MARRIED

Can't remember back that far. 73, WIDOWED

One time on New Year's Eve we timed our orgasm to be at midnight! 54, MARRIED

When I was 18, I went to a hotel with my boyfriend. Hotels are fun because they are different; you can make noise. And I was younger and had a stronger sex drive. 21, SINGLE

Still waiting. 73, WIDOWED

Now. It's uninhibited, no judgment. I finally know that men aren't that picky. 43, MARRIED

I was dressed to go out. Date arrives. He is turned on when he sees me. Sex on the sofa before we go out. It happened this year. 64, SINGLE

I hope I have not had it yet! 39, SINGLE

This year. I had sex with my ex-boyfriend on a conference room table in my office after hours. It was a combination of

the location being pretty risky and that we were completely comfortable with each other. 27, SINGLE

April 23, 2005, at age 63. It was the last time I had sex. 67, MARRIED

It's now. When I was younger, I was afraid to say what I liked during sex because of my cultural upbringing. I thought if I said I like certain things, a man would think I was a hoe. Now I realize men want to know and it makes them more into it. 35, MARRIED

I was 30-something. It was a quiet, almost desperate situation, with me wanting to comfort my husband on the loss of his mother. It was the only time we both had simultaneous orgasms. 52, WIDOWED

It was the first year of sex with my current husband. I was in my mid-thirties. At the time it was illicit, very wild. We lived out just about all of our fantasies in all sorts of places. It was incredibly memorable and I still fantastize about it. 49, MARRIED

WHAT IS THE BIGGEST LIE YOU WERE TOLD ABOUT SEX?

That it was easy to have an orgasm. 20, SINGLE

That intercourse alone is climactic. 55, MARRIED

A past lover claimed he surgically reduced the size of his penis. 73, MARRIED

That it gets better with age. 60, MARRIED

Other girls always want to have sex all of the time. 42, SINGLE

That being molested as a child would not affect my desire or outlook on sex. It did and does. 27, SINGLE

That men only want you for sex—made me think it was something I wouldn't enjoy. 49, MARRIED

That my vagina was nasty. (By my mother.) 49, MARRIED

That anal sex is pleasurable. 41, MARRIED

That sex stops in old age. 71, MARRIED

My mother told me sex was a store on Fifth Avenue. 82, MARRIED

That monogamy is the norm. 35, MARRIED

The nuns in catholic school told us if we had sex the devil would come into our rooms at night when everyone was asleep and beat us! 52, MARRIED

How great the experience is. I was never told about how sweaty and gross it can sometimes be. 26, SINGLE

That all women enjoy anal sex and have orgasms that way. 49, SINGLE

That it was my fault I wasn't enjoying it. 43, MARRIED

That you can lie in bed afterwards. It's too messy! 37, MARRIED

If the girl is on top, gravity pulls the sperm down. 15, SINGLE

That the first time is this great, enjoyable time. After it, I just thought, "Is that it?" 28, SINGLE

How great orgasms were—I only had one twice with men. Self stimulation produces orgasm most often. 71, MARRIED

Everyone can have a G-spot orgasm. SO many men have told me, "Oh you just haven't been with the right guy." Um, yes I have, and even he couldn't do it. 28, SINGLE

That sex is terrible, dirty and I'll go to hell if I do it.
63, DIVORCED

That it is better to have it a lot. Even when my (now long-distance) boyfriend and I lived together, we didn't do it a lot. We both feel it is much better if you wait a little. 22, SINGLE

That my husband alone would always be enough. I find sometimes we need the movies or toys to get things going.
34, MARRIED

That it would make things in a relationship better. Sex complicates everything. 19, SINGLE

That it hurt. Um .... NO. It's awesome! 22, SINGLE

United Parcel delivers babies. 60, MARRIED

Put the man first. 68, MARRIED

That 5 inches is 8 inches. 47, MARRIED

That I was frigid because my sex drive didn't match my husband's. He wanted it two or three times daily! 64, MARRIED

That you should wait until marriage. I only slept with two men and married them both. Now, at age 65, I wish I'd had more experiences. 65, MARRIED

Sex drive diminishes after menopause . . . wrong, wrong, wrong. 66, DIVORCED

That it's possible for everyone to have a simultaneous orgasm all the time like in a movie. 55, MARRIED

Bigger is better! NOT! 46, MARRIED

That you could get pregnant from a watermelon seed.
73, MARRIED

That you can't get pregnant if both you and your partner don't

have an orgasm at the same time. 40, SINGLE

That every time you have sex, you're supposed to come. 28, SINGLE

That you only have great sex if you love each other! 45, DIVORCED

Don't go in the dark with a boy or you can get pregnant. 66, DIVORCED

People make it seem that women have an orgasm all of the time, which is not true and in fact is very difficult for some of us. 18, SINGLE

That alcohol makes it better. Which is not the case. It makes you more willing, but does not make it better! 34, MARRIED

That sex and love are linked. 39, SINGLE

You don't get dirty. 54, MARRIED

That I would enjoy it more in my forties! 42, MARRIED

That my hysterectomy wouldn't change anything. 55, MAR-RIED

I promise not to come. 72, DIVORCED

ACKNOWLEDGMENTS

Anne Rodgers

A HEALTHY SUPPORT SYSTEM NOURISHES A WRITER, AND I AM blessed to have a strong one. Many dear friends offered kindness, expertise and encouragement during *Kiss and Tell's* lengthy timeline.

My partner and expert, Dr. Maureen Whelihan, was the original impetus; her relationship with her patients inspired this book, and her enthusiasm and resources never flagged as we waded into the unfamiliar world of publishing.

My deepest gratitude goes to each patient who agreed to talk about the intimate details of her sex life: They are the heart and soul of *Kiss and Tell.*

I thank my family for their encouragement, especially my mother who also lent a hand financially when things got tight.

I'm grateful to Chris Rothman for emotional guidance, to the Hershfields for the family love and to biking pal Ken Steinhoff for introducing me to cycling at the exact time I needed an escape from my desk. I offer heartfelt thanks as well to my talented writer friends who illuminated the way, particularly Sarah Bird, Scott Eyman and Hank Stuever.

My beta readers—Dianne King and Diane Porter—donated

innumerable hours of service, offering up their many years of professional experience out of pure friendship. Their input made *Kiss and Tell* immeasurably better.

Many devoted cheerleaders shouted encouragement along the way: Thanks Dorie, Patti, Marilyn and Bea! And Libby too, of course, whose sweet spirit saw me through some decidedly rough patches.

For the day-to-day hand holding and for the often-heavy work of lifting my spirits with encouraging words devoid of false assurance, all credit goes to Dianne King in Austin, Texas, my closest friend for more than half my life, and the one who never doubted.

Maureen Whelihan

I AM CONTINUALLY AMAZED AT THE HONESTY AND WILLING-ness of my patients to reveal their innermost secrets in order to help other women with similar concerns, and am grateful to all 1,300 women from my gynecology practice in West Palm Beach who participated in *Kiss and Tell*.

This project of passion took a team of committed enthusiasts who believed in getting the message out to women and men. This includes my office staff—Mary Compagnone, Patty Snow, Gail Camilleri and Becky Horvath—who encouraged participation from my patients at each visit.

Also, thanks to Judy Rosser, Jennifer Lowe, Gigi Naeve, Brittney Whelihan and numerous others who answered my call for opinions at various steps along the way. I am also grateful to my family—Gina Whelihan, Dave Whelihan, Joe Whelihan and my spouse, Cody Brown—who stayed committed to the project as if it was their own. Finally, my dad, David Whelihan Sr, who diligently counted all of the responses from the women and gave us a tally of the results. (Boy did he learn something—at 81 years old!)

Who knew we would learn so much in this lengthy endeavor? Because of Paul Joannides, I had some insight to the intense commitment of both time and energy. He was right on target with his predictions, and was an endless source of information and guidance.

Finally, thanks to my partner in this project—the superb writer, Anne Rodgers. What a wonderful team we make! Through her open and non-judgmental approach, her enthusiasm for understanding sexuality and her continual strive for clarity and perfection, we offer you our first project. Stay tuned for more to come!